KNOWLEDGE MEANS EMPOWERMENT.
TEST YOURSELF.

1. Can strenuous exercise cause your breasts to sag—or develop cancer?

2. How soon can a woman drop to pre-pregnancy weight after giving birth?

3. Which ethnic groups are at greatest risk for osteoporosis?

4. Do women athletes get injured more often than men?

5. Which two common professions for women hold significant, often overlooked risks during pregnancy?

6. Where, outside the home, are children at increased risk of lead poisoning?

ISN'T IT IMPORTANT THAT YOU HAVE THE FACTS? YOUR LIFE AND YOUR HEALTH MAY DEPEND ON IT.

Answers:

1. *No*
2. *18-20 pounds within 10 days after delivery; 2 pounds per month (if breast-feeding) afterward*
3. *Asian and white women*
4. *Two decades ago the answer was yes. With better training, injury rates have now dropped to the equivalent of men.*
5. *Nurses and hospital technicians*
6. *Playing near a busy street or in the soil around a painted home or building.*

Other books by the American Medical Women's Association

THE WOMEN'S COMPLETE HEALTHBOOK

The American Medical Women's Association

Guide to Nutrition and Wellness

Medical Co-editors
Roselyn Payne Epps, M.D., M.P.H., M.A., F.A.A.P.
Susan Cobb Stewart, M.D., F.A.C.P.

A Dell Book

Published by
Dell Publishing
a division of
Bantam Doubleday Dell Publishing Group, Inc.
1540 Broadway
New York, New York 10036

This material was originally published along with other material
in THE WOMEN'S COMPLETE HEALTHBOOK published by
Delacorte Press.

Illustrations by Wendy Frost

ISBN: 0-440-22244-3

Reprinted by arrangement with Delacorte Press

Printed in the United States of America

Published simultaneously in Canada

June 1996

10 9 8 7 6 5 4 3 2 1

OPM

The American Medical Women's Association

Guide to Nutrition and Wellness

THE AMWA GUIDE TO NUTRITION AND WELLNESS

Roselyn Payne Epps, M.D., M.P.H., M.A.,
and Susan Cobb Stewart, M.D.

Whether monitoring personal health care or the health care of immediate or extended families, women need a definitive source for accurate, dependable, and up-to-date information. *The AMWA Guide to Nutrition and Wellness* presents the essential components of overall good health as researched by the American Medical Women's Association (AMWA), the most historic and prestigious association of women physicians in the United States. Knowledge of physical, mental, and social concerns is crucial for detecting the early signs of many illnesses and for preventing potential diseases.

AMWA believes that women must avoid a disease-oriented approach to women's health and focus on maintaining optimal health on a daily and long-term basis. The more one knows about one's body and its functions, the better equipped one will be to safeguard good health through preventive strategies such as eating properly and exercising regularly. The content of *The AMWA Guide to Nutrition and Wellness* is organized into four major sections, each of which stresses the importance of preventive medicine and encourages total body awareness to avoid future health problems.

Part I, "Diet, Nutrition, and Healthy Weight," alerts the reader to nutritional issues that are important for women at various stages in their lives and during times of special requirements. It presents guidelines for a number of healthy diets for all women, including vegetarians, and discusses the importance of achieving the proper balance between nutritional intake, weight, and exercise. While being overweight can be dangerous to the heart, muscles, and bones, women need to be equally aware of the risks involved in being too thin, such as malnutrition and anorexia nervosa. This section cautions women against extreme weight of any kind and establishes guidelines for women to achieve their optimal weight based on factors such as age, body type, and life stage.

Part II, "Exercise and Physical Fitness," informs the reader of the importance of maintaining the proper balance between too little and too much exercise. It educates the reader to the fact that, when it comes to exercise, women have different training requirements and needs. Lack of exercise, for example, can cause health problems ranging from complicated pregnancy to a higher risk of cardiovascular disease. Regular exercise, on the other hand, enhances mood, stamina, appearance, and equilibrium, while reducing the risk of chronic diseases by keeping weight, blood fats, and sugars in check. Detailed in this section are the benefits and potential dangers of exercise, different types of fitness regimes, and methods of injury prevention.

Part III, "Living in a Healthy Environment," describes the health hazards around the home that can lead to health problems. In addition to the countless biological, chemical, and physical risks commonly found around the house, there are also many hidden dangers that directly threaten childbearing women, such as household plants and cat litter. This section will help you beware of potential hazards and to correct problems before they cause illness or injury.

Part IV, "Working in a Healthy Enviroment," addresses the needs of the increasing number of women who have entered the workforce. Some problems that disproportionately affect women are recognized only when women enter the labor force in substantial numbers. The book addresses the three major issues for women in the workplace: those based on size and shape differences, those concerning reproduction and pregnancy, and those stemming from social factors. A section on legal rights and resources identifies places where women workers can obtain counsel, legal advice, or join support groups to help cope with work-related problems.

The AMWA Guide to Nutrition and Wellness provides authoritative information that all women need in today's changing environment. It illuminates the health concerns unique to women of the 1990s and offers sound medical advice. Supported by the expertise and experience of the American Medical Women's Association, *The AMWA Guide to Nutrition and Wellness* is a progressive and comprehensive approach to health maintenance and wellness for women of all ages.

CONTENTS

PART 1
Diet, Nutrition, and Healthy Weight

Elaine B. Feldman, M.D., F.A.C.P

" **Y**ou are what you eat." Like many most popular phrases, this one has some merit. Everything that the body needs to function—from building materials for bones, muscles, and organs to the energy to run complex systems and processes—comes from and reflects the food and drink that make up our daily diet. Unhealthy diets lead to unhealthy bodies.

What is a healthy diet? New studies about the benefits and risks of eating certain foods are in the news nearly every day. It's difficult, though, to read between the lines and get the whole story. For example, huge quantities of a particular food may have had to be consumed for the reported results to take place. Or perhaps only a few people were studied, or the evidence was sketchy or preliminary. Some dietary habits are definitely linked to disease, however. We know that high levels of fat and cholesterol in the diet increase the risk of heart disease and stroke. Lack of fresh fruits and vegetables can promote disease, including cancer. On the other hand, a healthy diet can prevent disease and even ameliorate it.

GUIDELINES FOR A HEALTHY DIET

What makes a healthy diet? One of the best sets of recommendations is the U.S. government's *Dietary Guidelines for Americans*. Updated in 1990, these seven easy rules provide for a varied and well-balanced diet.

1. Eat a variety of foods.
2. Maintain healthy weight.
3. Choose a diet low in fat, saturated fat, and cholesterol.
4. Choose a diet with plenty of vegetables, fruits, and grain.
5. Use sugars only in moderation.
6. Use salt and sodium only in moderation.
7. If you drink alcoholic beverages, do so in moderation.

Women who make habits out of these seven guidelines will reduce their risk of disease, feel better, and live longer. It's never too soon—or too late—to start.

Guideline 1: Eat a Variety of Foods

Different foods are good sources of different nutrients. By eating a varied diet, you increase your chances of getting all the nutrients your body needs. Plus, eating many different foods makes dinnertime a lot more interesting. The problem is choosing which foods to eat for basic health maintenance.

Choosing from Food Groups

You may remember learning about the "Four Food Groups" in school. There were four categories: milk and dairy products, meat and protein foods, fruits and vegetables, and grains and cereals. Unfortunately, this grouping seems to put too much emphasis on the first two categories. Most Americans get more protein in their diets than they may need, and dairy products and meats are high in fat.

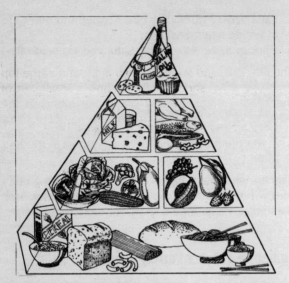

Figure 1.1 The Food Guide Pyramid.

In 1992, the U.S. Department of Agriculture introduced the "Food Guide Pyramid" as a way to give Americans a better guide to food selection (Figure 1.1). More servings per day are recommended of the foods at the bottom of the pyramid, and fewer servings per day are needed of those at the top. The pyramid is divided into the following basic food categories:

1. Bread, cereal, rice, and pasta (6 to 11 servings per day)
2. Vegetables (3 to 5 servings per day)
3. Fruit (2 to 4 servings per day)

4. Meat, poultry, fish, dry beans, eggs, and nuts (2 to 3 servings per day)
5. Milk, yogurt, and cheese (2 to 3 servings per day)

The fats, oils, and sweets, which are found at the top of the pyramid, should make up only a small part of the healthy diet. Fats and sugars are found in the other groups of the pyramid, too. Some occur naturally, such as the sugars in fruit or the fats in meat or milk. Others are added, such as the fats and sugars in baked goods.

You should eat foods from each group on a daily basis. How many calories you need each day depends on your age, your size, how active you are, and whether you are pregnant or breast-feeding. Here is a general guide:

- Women who get little exercise and small older women: 1,600 calories per day

- Most children, teenage girls, and active women (women who are pregnant or breast-feeding may need more): 2,000 or more calories per day

- Very active women: 2,400 or more calories per day

Once you know about how many calories you need, you can choose the right number of servings from each food group (Table 1.1).

Serving sizes are important, too. If serving sizes are too big, even of nutritious food, the extra calories may lead to weight gain. If too small, the foods may not provide all of the needed nutrients. Table 1.2 gives examples of serving sizes for each food group.

TABLE 1.1 CHOOSING THE RIGHT NUMBER OF SERVINGS

Food Group	1,600 Calories	2,200 Calories	2,800 Calories
Breads (servings)	6	9	11
Vegetables (servings)	3	4	5
Fruits (servings)	2	3	4
Dairy products* (servings)	2	2	2
Meats (ounces)	5	6	7

Source: Modified from the U.S. Department of Agriculture, *The Food Guide Pyramid* (Home and Garden Bulletin No. 252), Washington, D.C.: USDA, 1992.

*Women who are pregnant or breast-feeding, teenagers, and young adults (up to age 24) need 3 servings of dairy products per day.

Nutrients

Nutrients are the basic components of food. Nutrients fall into six categories: proteins, carbohydrates, fats, vitamins, minerals, and water. All of these are a part of a healthy diet, but the body needs more of some nutrients and less of others.

Proteins

Proteins are the building blocks of the body. They form muscles and organs and are responsible for the repair and maintenance of tissues. Some hormones, especially the polypeptide type like insulin, are made from amino acids. Important as they are, only about 15 percent of the calories in the average woman's diet

TABLE 1.2   WHAT COUNTS AS A SERVING?

Food Group	Serving Size
Breads	• 1 slice of bread • 1 ounce of ready-to-eat cereal • $^1/_2$ cup of cooked cereal, rice, or pasta
Vegetables	• 1 cup of raw leafy vegetables • $^1/_2$ cup of other vegetables, cooked or chopped raw • $^3/_4$ cup of vegetable juice
Fruits	• 1 medium apple, banana, or orange • $^1/_2$ cup of chopped, cooked, or canned fruit • $^3/_4$ cup of fruit juice
Dairy products	• 1 cup of milk or yogurt • $1^1/_2$ ounces of natural cheese • 2 ounces of process cheese
Meats	• 2 to 3 ounces of cooked lean meat, poultry, or fish • $^1/_2$ cup of cooked dry beans • 1 egg • 2 tablespoons of peanut butter

Source: U.S. Department of Agriculture, The Food Guide Pyramid (Home and Garden Bulletin No. 252), Washington, D.C.: USDA, 1992.

must come from proteins.

Animal foods, such as meats and milk, are good sources of complete protein. A complete protein contains all of the *essential amino acids* our bodies need. Amino acids are the building blocks of proteins, and essential amino acids are the ones that we must obtain from our diets because our bodies cannot

READING LABELS

Recent federal regulations require that all labels on packaged foods provide information on the number of calories and amount of fat, saturated fat, cholesterol, sodium, carbohydrates, dietary fiber, sugar, and protein that food contains. The information is related to a normal daily diet that contains 2,000 calories, 65 grams of fat (30 percent of calories), 20 grams of saturated fat, 300 milligrams of cholesterol, 2,400 milligrams of sodium, 300 grams of total carbohydrates, and 25 grams of fiber. The percentage of the daily values that one serving of the food provides is given, along with a percentage of the daily value for vitamin A, vitamin C, calcium, and iron.

Use the information on food labels to limit the amount of your fat consumption. Here's how to find the percentage of calories from fat in one serving of a food:

1.   Multiply the number of grams of fat in a serving, as shown on the label, by 9 (there are 9 calories in each gram of fat) to find the number of calories from fat.

2.   Divide the number of calories from fat by the total number of calories, on the label, shown for one serving.

3.   Multiply this amount by 100 to get the percentage of calories from fat.

If you look at any package label, you will see that one serving of pretzels has 1.5 grams of total fat and 180 calories. (1) The total number of calories from fat is 1.5 × 9, or about 14 calories from fat. (Total calories from fat is often shown on food labels.) (2) Divide 14 by 180 (the number of calories in one serving), which comes to 0.077. (3) Finally, multiply by 100. About 8 percent of the calories in these pretzels come from fat.

Be alert to serving sizes, which are also listed on the label. If the label specifies two cookies as one serving, and you eat four cookies, you'll need to multiply all of the nutritional information by two to get the nutrient content of the food you consumed.

Fresh meat, fish, poultry, and produce are not required to carry labels with this information. Sometimes this information is available at the produce or meat counter of grocery stores.

manufacture them. Proteins are found in plants as well. Legumes are a particularly good source of plant protein. Legumes are beans and peas such as kidney beans, lentils, soybeans, garbanzo beans (chick-peas), and black-eyed peas. Grains, such as corn and wheat, are also good sources of plant protein. Different types of plants have different amino acids. Thus vegetarians can get enough of the essential amino acids if they eat the appropriate variety of plant proteins.

Carbohydrates

Carbohydrates come in two kinds: simple and complex. Simple carbohydrates, or sugars, are easily digested by the body and provide a source of quick energy. Complex carbohydrates, or starches, are made up of long chains of molecules, and provide long-lasting energy and dietary fiber. Breads, pasta, grains, cereals, and some vegetables are complex carbohydrates. Carbohydrates should make up at least 55 percent of the calories in the average woman's diet.

Fats

Fats are the four-letter word of the nutrition world, but they do serve a purpose—in small quantities. A certain amount of fat is vital to maintaining good health, and fats are packed with energy (and calories). While proteins and carbohydrates contain 4 calories per gram (31 grams equal 1 ounce), fats have more than twice as many calories per gram—9 in all. Fats help the body absorb the so-called fat-soluble vitamins. Because of their tendency to raise blood cholesterol levels, fats should make up no more than 30 percent of the calories in the average woman's diet, and saturated fats—those that solidify at room temperature—should make up no more than 10 percent. Saturated fats include butter, hard cheese, the fats from beef and other meats and the vegetable fats of coconut, palm kernel, and palm oils.

Vitamins and Minerals

Vitamins are organic substances that are essential to a wide variety of body functions, including the biochemical conversion of protein, carbohydryates, and fats into energy. Minerals are inorganic substances that help control many metabolic processes. The body needs both vitamins and minerals to realize its full potential. The Recommended Dietary Allowances (RDAs) issued by the U.S. government show how much of each nutrient the average healthy woman needs (Table 1.3). Women who are pregnant or breast-feeding have special needs and require more of some nutrients in their diet.

Different foods contain different amounts of vitamins and minerals, so consuming a variety of foods is the best way to get all these nutrients (Table 1.4). Some commercial foods are enriched to provide more nutrients, including white flour, cereals, and pasta. Fruit juices may have added calcium, and vitamin D is usually added to milk. To preserve vitamin value, do not overcook foods, especially vegetables.

Vitamin and mineral supplements may benefit some women. If you are pregnant or breast-feeding or if you are a vegetarian, you may have special needs or dietary inadequacies that can only be met by supplements. Note that consuming large amounts of some vitamins and minerals may be dangerous, however; and there are few proven health benefits to "megadosing." Therefore, do not take much more than is suggested by the RDAs. This is especially true of vitamins A and D, which are fat soluble and stored in the body. Consuming too much of vitamins A and D can poison the body. Therapeutic or high-potency vitamins may have two to three times the RDAs for the B vitamins and vitamin C. They may be helpful if you have had recent illness, weight loss, or surgery.

TABLE 1.3 RECOMMENDED DIETARY ALLOWANCES FOR WOMEN

Nutrient	Nonpregnant (years old)					Pregnant	Breast-Feeding
	15 to 18	19 to 24	25 to 50	50	51+		
Protein (grams)	44	46	50	50	50	60	65
Vitamins							
Vitamin A (micrograms)	800	800	800	800	800	800	1,300
Vitamin B₁* (milligrams)	1.1	1.1	1.1	1.1	1.0	1.5	1.6
Vitamin B₂† (milligrams)	1.3	1.3	1.3	1.3	1.2	1.6	1.8
Vitamin B₃‡ (milligrams)	15	15	15	15	13	17	20
Vitamin B₆§ (milligrams)	1.5	1.6	1.6	1.6	1.6	2.2	2.1
Vitamin B₁₂|| (micrograms)	2	2	2	2	2	2.2	2.6
Vitamin C (milligrams)	60	60	60	60	60	70	95
Vitamin D (micrograms)	10	10	5	5	5	10	10
Vitamin E (milligrams)	8	8	8	8	8	10	12
Vitamin K (micrograms)	55	60	65	65	65	65	65
Folic acid (micrograms)	180	180	180	180	180	400	280

Minerals

Calcium (milligrams)	1,200	1,200	800	800#	1,200	1,200
Iodine (micrograms)	150	150	150	150	175	200
Iron (milligrams)	15	15	15	10	30	15
Magnesium (milligrams)	300	280	280	280	320	355
Phosphorus (milligrams)	1,200	1,200	800	800	1,200	1,200
Selenium (micrograms)	50	55	55	55	65	75
Zinc (milligrams)	12	12	12	12	15	19

Source: Adapted from National Academy of Sciences, *Recommended Dietary Allowances,* Washington, D.C.: National Academy Press, 1989.

* Thiamin.
† Riboflavin.
‡ Niacin.
§ Pyridoxine.
‖ Cobalamin.
Some medical authorities recommend 1,500 milligrams.

TABLE 1.4   SOME VITAMINS AND MINERALS

Nutrient	Function in Body
Vitamins	
Vitamin A	Needed for normal vision in dim light; prevents eye diseases; needed for growth of bones and teeth
Vitamin B_1 (thiamin)	Helps body digest carbohydrates; needed for normal functioning of nervous system
Vitamin B_2 (riboflavin)	Helps body release energy to cells; promotes healthy skin and eyes
Vitamin B_3 (niacin)	Promotes healthy skin, nerves, and digestion; helps the body use carbohydrates
Vitamin B_6 (pyridoxine)	Helps form red blood cells; helps body use protein, fat, and carbohydrate
Vitamin B_{12} (cobalamin)	Maintains nervous system; needed to form red blood cells
Vitamin C	Speeds healing of wounds and bones; increases resistance to infection; needed to form collagen
Vitamin D*	Helps body use calcium and phosphorus; needed for strong bones and teeth
Vitamin E	Needed for use of vitamin A; helps body form and use red blood cells and muscles
Vitamin K	Aids in making blood-clotting factors
Folic acid	Needed to produce blood cells and protein; helps some enzymes function
Minerals	
Calcium	Needed for strong bones and teeth; helps in blood clotting; needed for normal muscle and nerve function
Iodine	Needed to produce thyroid hormones that regulate body's energy use
Iron	Needed to make hemoglobin; prevents anemia; increases resistance to infection
Magnesium	Needed for nerve and muscle function; helps body use carbohydrates
Phosphorus	Needed for strong bones and teeth
Selenium	Prevents breakdown of body chemicals
Zinc	Needed to produce some enzymes and insulin

* Also manufactured in the body when the skin is exposed to ultraviolet radiation (sunlight).

Diet Source

Liver, fish liver oils, butter, carrots, spinach, cantaloupe, sweet potatoes

Enriched or whole-grain cereals, pastas, peas, nuts, beans, meats

Liver, milk, yogurt, cottage cheese, eggs, leafy vegetables

Liver, peanuts, chicken, salmon, tuna

Liver, meat, fish, poultry, peanuts

Liver, meat, eggs, shellfish

Citrus fruits, melons, strawberries, green pepper, broccoli, brussels sprouts, turnip greens

Fortified milk, fish liver oils, fish, egg yolks

Vegetable oils, margarine, meat, peas, nuts

Green tea, turnip greens, broccoli, leafy vegetables

Liver, leafy vegetables, oranges, peanuts

Milk, cheese, sardines (with bones), tortillas, almonds, broccoli and other green vegetables

Seafood (haddock, cod, lobster), iodized salt, dairy products, bread

Meat, calves' liver, poultry, fish, beans, raisins

Milk, meats, seafood, cereal, peanuts, bananas, dark green leafy vegetables

Milk, bologna, liver, hamburger, cheese

Seafood, organ meats, muscle meats, whole grains

Red meat, shellfish (oysters), eggs

Source: Data in columns 1 and 3 from E. B. Feldman, *Essentials of Clinical Nutrition,* Philadelphia: F. A. Davis, 1988. Data in column 2 from American College of Obstetricians and Gynecologists, *Planning for Pregnancy, Birth, and Beyond,* Washington, D.C.: ACOG, 1990.

CHOOSING AND PREPARING FOODS SAFELY

Natural foods and organic foods generally do not have special nutritional value. They also are more expensive than foods grown by commercial methods. Fertilizers used on commercially grown foods contain chemicals similar to those that appear in manure (used in organic farming) and the soil and plants themselves.

Pesticides are found on many foods, but the amounts present are usually very small. The U.S. government sets allowable limits for pesticide residues in food, and in 1987, only 1 percent of the food products sampled had residues higher than the limits. To limit your exposure to pesticides, make sure you wash vegetables and fruits thoroughly before eating them.

To prevent foodborne infections, handle certain foods and kitchen tools with care. Store raw meat, poultry, and fish separately from cooked foods or foods that will be eaten raw. Wash your hands well after handling raw meats, poultry, and fish and before working with other foods. Thoroughly wash cutting boards and surfaces used to prepare raw meats. For added protection, wipe cutting boards and countertops with a watered-down bleach.

Cook meats thoroughly, especially ground meat. Cook poultry until the juices run clear.

Fish should be cooked until it is translucent; overcooking will cause a loss of flavor. It is not recommended that you eat raw fish, because it may harbor parasites. Use products by their expiration date or freeze them for later use.

The proper storage of food is also important. Do not leave cooked foods at room temperature for long periods of time. Bacteria can multiply and toxins can form that will be present in the food, even if reheated. Refrigerate leftovers promptly.

However, in most cases, you should get the bulk of your vitamins and minerals from the food you eat.

Guideline 2: Maintain a Healthy Weight

Today women are bombarded by advertisements and the media to cultivate a slim waist, slender legs, and shapely breasts. The attainment of this "ideal" figure is generally unrealistic, and often downright unhealthy. But it is important that you maintain a healthy weight—one that is right for your age, size, and body structure. Not only will you look and feel better but you will reduce your risk of disease, particularly diabetes, heart disease, and hypertension.

Remember, being a few pounds overweight is not the same thing as being obese. Obesity means being more than 20 percent over your optimum weight. Where you carry the weight matters, too. Muscles weigh more than fat. If you are large and muscular, you may not have much body fat and may weigh more than recommended for your height and age, but this is not unhealthy. If you do have excess fat, note where it is stored in your body. Fat carried around the hips and thighs—the so-called pear shape—is considered to be less of a health risk than the apple shape—the big belly look seen in men and some women. The apple shape has been linked to heart disease, high blood pressure, and diabetes.

How Obesity Affects the Body

Too much poundage increases your risk of heart disease and hypertension. In fact, heart disease occurs two to three times more often in obese women than in women of normal weight. One reason for this is that many obese women have high levels of cholesterol in their blood. Cholesterol, a fatty substance, clogs the blood vessels, eventually causing a heart attack. Strokes are also more likely to occur if you

---

HEALTH RISKS OF OBESITY

If you are 20 percent or more over the recommended weight for your age, height, and body frame, you run the risk of developing

High blood pressure
Cardiovascular disease
Stroke
Diabetes
Arthritis (hips, knees, and ankles)
Gallstones
Cancer (uterine, breast, colon, and ovarian)

have high cholesterol levels. Women who are obese are more likely to have a sedentary lifestyle and high blood presssure, both of which raise the risk for cardiovascular disease.

The obese are more likely to have the most common type of diabetes, which is the inability of the body to metabolize sugar properly. Other risks of obesity include varicose veins; bloodclots in the legs; arthritis in the knees; gallbladder disease; hernias; breathing problems; and cancers of the uterus, breast, colon, and rectum.

What Is a Healthy Weight?

A healthy weight depends on several factors: your height, your body frame size, and your age. Taller women, women with larger bone structures, and older women have higher weight allowances. Table 1.5 lists recommended body weights based on height and age. Another way to calculate the suggested weight for a given height is the body mass index (BMI) (see "Calculating Your BMI").

Controlling Your Weight

The United States is fortunate in that it has an abundance of available food and its population is one of the best fed in the world. Malnutrition certainly exists in our society, but the greater problem is obesity. Unfortunately, there is much confusion in the public perception of body image—women who are only minimally overweight struggle to lose weight, while many obese women, tired of dieting, give up and decide to live with their problem, however severe.

Women who are greatly overweight or obese can

improve their health and lower their risk of disease by rejecting calorie-counting diets and by sticking to a sensible plan of weight control. Weight control means not only losing pounds but keeping the pounds off. Permanent weight loss, then, requires a change in lifestyle and a new attitude toward food and eating. It means not thinking in terms of "dieting"

TABLE 1.5 USDA SUGGESTED WEIGHTS FOR WOMEN*

Height	Age	
	19 to 34 years	**>35 years**
60"	97–128	108–138
61"	101–132	111–143
62"	104–137	115–148
63"	107–141	119–152
64"	111–146	122–157
65"	114–150	126–162
66"	118–155	130–167
67"	121–160	134–172
68"	125–164	138–178
69"	129–169	142–183
70"	132–174	146–188
71"	136–179	151–194
72"	140–184	155–199

Source: American College of Obstetricians and Gynecologists, *Weight Control: Eating Right and Keeping Fit* (ACOG Patient Education Pamphlet AP064), Washington, D.C.: ACOG, 1993.

* Height, in inches, is without shoes. Weight, in pounds, is without clothes. The lower weights more often apply to women who have less muscle and bone.

at all. Dieting is merely a temporary restriction of all your favorite foods, which comes to an end as soon as a particular weight goal is met. Making permanent changes certainly is more difficult, but the benefits pay off for a lifetime. These changes include focusing on the right foods, engaging in regular exercise, and perhaps finding the right support system.

CALCULATING YOUR BMI

You can calculate your body mass index (BMI) by using the following formula:

$$\frac{\text{Weight (in kilograms)}}{\text{Height (in meters) squared}}$$

To convert your weight and height to metrics, note that 1 pound is equal to 0.45 kilogram and 1 inch is equal to 0.0254 meter. For example, a woman who weighs 120 pounds and is 64 inches tall also weighs 54 kilograms (120 × 0.45) and is 1.63 meters tall (64 × 0.0254). Her BMI would be 54 ÷ (1.63 × 1.63), or about 20.3, which puts her in the normal range. Normal, overweight, and obese ranges for BMIs vary, but in general, a BMI of 20 to 25 is considered normal, 25 to 30 is considered overweight, and over 30 is considered obese. Using these ranges, up to 33 percent of the U.S. population should be considered obese. Obesity is more common in women than in men.

Dietary Changes

A sensible plan for weight loss means losing about 0.5 to 1 pound a week. More rapid weight loss may be achieved by starvation-type diets, but these regimens don't work in the long run. Furthermore, there are physiological reasons for the failure of most of these kinds of diets. When the body suddenly stops taking in the accustomed amount of calories, it acts as though it were starving. The rate of metabolism, or how fast your body burns the calories needed to maintain daily functions, slows down. If the diet is still restricted, weight loss occurs slowly if at all (the so-called plateau of dieting). The dieter becomes discouraged and may begin to sneak in some extra calories. After the weight is gained back, she begins dieting again. This on-again, off-again *yo-yo* dieting is counterproductive—the weight is gained back rapidly, and each time a new diet starts, the body's metabolism slows down still more. The pounds are harder to lose each time you try.

Generally, reputable plans for weight loss do not restrict calories to less than 1,200 a day. On a sensible lifetime plan, foods can be chosen from all the food groups. There is even room for most of your favorite snacks—including chocolate—if portions are kept small and the fat content is minimal (Table 1.6). The best plans emphasize a gradual weight loss that, ideally, is combined with a real desire to make changes that will eventually become part and parcel of a new, healthier lifestyle.

TABLE 1.6 EATING SENSIBLY

Food Group	Choose More Often	Choose Less Often
Breads	Whole-grain breads; whole-grain and bran cereals; rice; pasta	Refined-flour breads and cakes; biscuits; croissants; crackers; chips; cookies; pastries; granola
Vegetables	Dark green, leafy vegetables (spinach, collard, endive); yellow-orange vegetables (carrots, sweet potatoes, squash); cabbage; broccoli; cauliflower; brussels sprouts	Avocados; vegetables prepared in butter, oil, and cream sauces
Fruits	Citrus fruits (oranges, grapefruit); apples; berries; pears	Coconut; fruit pies; pastries
Dairy products	Low-fat or skim milk; low-fat or nonfat yogurt and cheeses (ricotta, farmer, cottage, mozzarella); sherbet; frozen low-fat yogurt; ice milk	Whole milk; butter; yogurt made from whole milk; sweet cream, sour cream, whipped cream, and other creamy toppings (including imitation); ice cream; coffee creamers (including nondairy); cream cheese; cheese spreads; Brie; Camembert; hard cheeses (Swiss, Cheddar)
Meats	Low-fat chicken or turkey (white meat without skin); fresh or frozen fish; water-packed canned tuna; lean meat trimmed of all fat; cooked dry beans and peas; egg whites and egg substitutes	Beef, veal, lamb, and pork cuts with marbling, untrimmed of fat; duck; goose; organ meats; luncheon meats; sausage; hot dogs; peanut butter; nuts; seeds; trail mix; tuna packed in oil; egg yolks; whole eggs

Source: Adapted from American College of Obstetricians and Gynecologists, *Cholesterol and Your Health* (ACOG Patient Education Pamphlet 101), Washington, D.C.: ACOG, 1993.

Exercise

Regular exercise not only burns fat but also helps raise the body's metabolic rate, and it increases the size and tone of the muscles. In addition, regular exercise increases your overall fitness and improves your sense of well-being and self-esteem.

Because regular exercise is so essential, it is important to choose a workout that you enjoy and will pursue often. Choose some activity that is convenient and readily accessible. Although downhill skiing can be fun and is great for burning calories, it's difficult for most women to build a regular exercise program around skiing. Instead, choose jogging, brisk walking, swimming, biking, or aerobic dancing as the core of your exercise program, with other sports added for fun.

Aerobic exercise works the heart and lungs, and it is the best exercise for weight control and overall fitness. Your workout should up your heart rate into your target heart rate zone (Table 1.7). The target heart rate is 60 to 80 percent of your maximum heart rate. (You can determine your maximum heart rate by subtracting your age from 220.) After checking with your doctor, start slowly, aiming for the low end of your target heart rate zone. Exercise three times a week for 20 to 30 minutes at a time. As you become more fit, you can work out every day for 45 to 60 minutes at a time.

Weight Loss Support

Although most women who lose weight successfully do so on their own, some of us need guidance and support. There are many professionals and organizations who can help you in your weight loss ven-

TABLE 1.7 TARGET HEART RATE

Age (years)	Beats per Minute
20	120–160
25	117–156
30	114–152
35	111–148
40	108–144
45	105–140
50	102–136
55	99–132
60	96–128
65	93–124
70	90–120

Source: Adapted from National Heart, Lung, and Blood Institute, *Exercise and Your Heart* (NIH Publication No. 81-1677), Washington, D.C.: U.S. Government Printing Office, 1981.

ture. Doctors and nutritionists can plan a weight loss program or refer you to a reputable organization. Many commercial weight loss programs may be a good source of education and support. Weight Watchers and Overeaters Anonymous are two well-known programs. University-based health or wellness programs also exist. If you are interested in joining a weight loss program, do some reseach. Find out how each program operates, what type of weight loss it recommends, and how much it costs. Some programs require that participants purchase some or all of their food from the program. This may seem convenient, but these foods are usually more expensive than similar foods purchased in the grocery store or cooked at

DIETARY MYTHS

The most common dietary myths relate to food and its effects. Books, magazines, and TV talk shows are prime sources of the latest food fads, usually for losing weight. Some fad diets promise quick results, which don't last. Other fad diets are so unbalanced that they could actually harm your health if prolonged. The cruelest food hoaxes are those aimed at persons who have cancer or other serious diseases. Women who believe that concoctions of peach pits can cure their cancer will *not* benefit from such treatment, and they may delay seeking medical care early, when their conditions are most treatable.

Remember, if something sounds too good to be true, it probably is. Watch out for these dietary myths:

- Starchy foods are especially fattening.
- Cottage cheese and grapefruit are slimming.
- Special wraps, lotions, and pills can promote weight loss.
- Some diets, like the extremes of the Zen macrobiotic diet, carry no serious health risks.
- Tests for nutritional status based on hair analysis (or other unorthodox strategies) are sound and accurate.

- Taking tryptophan is a safe way to relieve insomnia.
- Vitamin C prevents colds.
- Special foods promote sexuality or act as a "fountain of youth."
- Some special foods or vitamins can cure cancer or mental illness.

home. Relying on a preplanned diet of special foods can also make it difficult for you to maintain your weight loss after you reach your ideal weight. Learning to choose foods wisely is a vital part of remaking one's lifstyle, and this important skill may not be learned as readily in programs that rely on special foods.

Women who are severely obese need more than supportive programs to lose weight. They need medical help. Weight loss programs for severely obese women should be developed and monitored by a doctor or nurse.

Eating Disorders

It's dangerous to be overweight, but it's also risky to eat and weigh too little. Some women, especially teenage girls, have a distorted image of their bodies. Even if their weight is normal, they may see themselves as grossly overweight and may embark on strict diets and rigorous exercise programs. These women may be suffering from an eating disorder that can have grave effects on their health, both physically and psychologically.

Particularly devastating is *anorexia nervosa*, a

chronic eating disorder. Women with anorexia, no matter what their weight, believe they are overweight and severely cut down on the amount of food they eat. Sometimes these women starve themselves to the point of emaciation. They also may exercise to extremes, led on by their pathological fear of gaining weight. Teenagers as well as models, gymnasts, dancers, and long-distance runners are at risk for this serious condition, which can lead to severe malnutrition, even death.

Binge eating, or *bulimia,* is closely associated with anorexia. Women with bulimia eat huge amounts of high-calorie foods—usually sweets—at one sitting, and then undergo self-induced vomiting so they won't gain weight. Many of these women use laxatives or diuretics to force fluids quickly out of their systems. This overuse of medications can seriously disrupt the body's chemical balance and increase the chances of heart problems, including fatal arrythmias. Like anorexia, bulimia can lead to death. Unlike women with anorexia, however, women suffering from bulimia recognize that their eating habits are abnormal. They often become severely depressed after a bulimic episode and may seek help more quickly than do women with anorexia.

There is a strong psychological compulsion connected with these illnesses, and both medical and psychological help is necessary to treat them successfully. Treatment may be long term, as it can take some time to relearn healthy patterns of eating.

Guideline 3: Choose a Diet Low in Fat, Saturated Fat, and Cholesterol

A healthy diet includes reducing your fat intake to 30 percent or less of your total daily calories. Keep in mind that saturated fat—the kind of fat that is solid at room temperature—has the worst effect on the blood cholesterol. However, it is important to note that cholesterol levels in the blood are not 100 percent diet related: There is also a genetic component at work. Some women have low cholesterol no matter what they eat, while others have high levels of cholesterol despite a low-fat diet.

The Health Risks of a High Fat Diet

There is a strong association between diet and the development of heart disease and cancer. The consumption of too much fat may increase the risk of developing these diseases, but other foods may actually reduce your risk.

Heart Disease

Cardiac problems are the leading causes of death for American women. Heart disease tends to occur later in women than it does in men, presumably because premenopausal women produce estrogen, a hormone that seems to provide some protection against heart disease. The level of estrogen, however, drops drastically at menopause, when menstrual periods stop. Without the protection of estrogen, a woman's risk of heart disease begins to climb.

If you consume high levels of saturated fat and cholesterol, sticky lumps may build up in your arteries, leading to a condition called *atherosclerosis*. Eventually, the arteries may clot off or become completely blocked, causing a stroke or heart attack.

Not all blood cholesterol is bad, however. When you consume fat, it is digested and bound into fatty packages called lipoproteins. Lipoproteins carry the fat through the blood vessels for use or storage in other parts of the body. There are three main types of lipoproteins:

- Very low-density lipoproteins (VLDLs)
- Low-density lipoproteins (LDLs)
- High-density lipoproteins (HDLs)

The VLDLs carry fat and cholesterol through the bloodstream to fat tissue. After they drop off some of the fat, they become LDLs. LDLs are sometimes called carriers of "bad cholesterol" because this type of cholesterol builds up in the blood vessels. HDLs are called "good cholesterol" particles because they pick up the cholesterol that has been deposited in the blood vessels and carry it back to the liver where the body can get rid of the cholesterol. Trouble arises when there is not enough good HDL to carry the LDL cholesterol deposits away. To keep down the level of your LDLs, choose a low-fat low-cholesterol diet. Exercise increases the amount of HDLs in your body, another reason why it's important to exercise regularly.

Cancer
A diet high in fats seems to increase the risk of some cancers, although the exact reasons for this are unknown. In particular, a high-fat, high-calorie diet is believed to increase the risk of cancer of the breast,

uterus, colon, and ovaries. One theory postulates that fats may increase a woman's production of some estrogen products that promote cancer. While estrogen does help prevent heart disease, too much estrogen is believed to be a prime cause of reproductive cancer in older women. Some authorities recommend a diet of less than 20 percent of calories from fat to reduce the risk of breast cancer.

Finding and Preparing the Right Foods

Today, it is easier than ever to make low-fat foods part of a delicious, healthy diet. From nonfat ice cream to crackers and cookies, low-fat foods are a major growth industry in this country. Restaurants, too, have gotten on the low-fat bandwagon (see "Eating Out").

When shopping, read food labels carefully, especially noting when a product is called "low-fat" or "90 percent fat-free." These claims may not reflect the true calories from fat in the food. The problem with figuring the percentage of fat in a product is that the percentage is based on weight, including water. For example, ground meat is about 70 percent water. So, even if the meat is labeled "10 percent fat by weight," it still derives over 50 percent of its calories from fat.

As with other types of dietary changes, the key word in reducing fat intake is *moderation*. Drastic changes in the diet are much more difficult to accept and maintain. Instead, adopt the concept of choosing low-fat foods more often and high-fat foods less often. Limit the use of saturated fats in general, and use vegetable oils such as olive and canola oils. Watch the portion size of protein-rich foods. You only need about 6 ounces for the entire day. Vegetables

EATING OUT

When newspaper articles report on the high amount of fat in Chinese, Italian, and Mexican foods, you may think it's impossible to find a low-fat restaurant meal. Just as at home, though, healthy meals can be had by selecting low-fat options and avoiding the high-fat items.

- At Chinese restaurants, eat more rice and vegetables and less meat and sauce. Skip the fried appetizers and choose steamed dumplings or soup instead.

- At Italian restaurants, select pastas with tomato-based sauces instead of pastas topped with heavy cream and cheese sauces. Pick a salad (with dressing on the side) instead of garlic bread.

- At Mexican restaurants, rice and beans, if not refried in fat, are a healthy part of your meal. Chicken soft tacos and fajitas are acceptable too. Skip the fried taco shells and taco salads, and limit your intake of sour cream, cheese, and guacamole.

- At fast-food restaurants, choose a plain burger over one with the works, and hold the cheese. Grilled chicken sandwiches are a good choice if not breaded. Try a salad bar instead of fries, but keep the portion reasonable and choose raw vegetables instead of prepared pasta or bean salads.

and grains (starches) are filling and low in fat, so make them the center of a meal, and use protein-rich foods for accent. Instead of red meat, choose chicken (without skin), fish (fish oil may help protect against heart disease), and plant proteins (such as peas and beans).

Many of your favorite foods can be easily adapted to provide the same flavors with lower calories. Try making salad dressings with a tomato or yogurt base instead of oil or mayonnaise. Nonfat yogurt can substitute for high-fat sour cream. Milk shakes can be made with fruit and nonfat frozen yogurt or ice milk. Try an angel food cake instead of a layer cake.

Be alert to methods of food preparation, too. Avoid frying, or pan fry in a skillet sprayed with a nonstick vegetable oil. Grilling, broiling, and microwaving are good low-fat methods for cooking meats, poultry, and fish.

Guideline 4: Choose a Diet with Plenty of Vegetables, Fruits, and Grains

As shown in the Food Guide Pyramid (see Fig. 1.1), vegetables, fruits, and grains are the foundation of a healthy diet. Fortunately, these foods are inexpensive and an excellent source of vitamins, minerals, and fiber. Fiber helps the body feel full, improves bowel function, and also seems to protect against cancers of the colon and rectum. Vegetables, fruits, and grains are naturally low in fat and sodium and contain no cholesterol.

Try to build meals around these healthy foods

and go easier on dairy and meat products. Vegetable soup, whole-grain bread, and a salad, for instance, make a great low-fat meal that is loaded with fiber, vitamins, and minerals.

Guideline 5: Use Sugar Only in Moderation

Foods high in sugar tend to have *empty calories*— calories without other nutrients. Besides adding calories, sugar may also take the place of healthy foods in the diet and prevent you from getting all the nutrients you need. Digested rapidly by the body, sugar provides a quick energy source that may be used up just as quickly. Consuming complex starches instead provides a more even, longer-lasting energy source. Finally, foods high in sugar, especially sticky sweets, promote tooth decay.

Try making healthy substitutions when the sweet tooth strikes. Fruit or fruit juice is a healthy option, for example. If you do indulge in an occasional dessert, keep the portion small. Cereals, processed foods, and baked goods are often high in hidden sugars, so check the label before buying. Another tip: Put fruit on your breakfast cereal instead of sugar.

Guideline 6: Use Salt Only in Moderation

The average American diet is too high in salt—over 9 grams a day. Your daily salt intake should be no more than 6 grams ($1^1/_2$ teaspoons). Sodium can increase blood pressure in susceptible people. A few studies have indicated that sensitivity to salt increases with age, so get in the habit now of moderating your salt intake. Try to avoid using salt when cooking or at the table. Instead, use herbs and other spices to perk up a dish. Many processed foods are high in sodium, so check labels before buying. Some manufacturers now offer products containing low or no sodium.

Guideline 7: If You Drink Alcoholic Beverages, Do So in Moderation

Women who use alcohol should limit their daily intake to no more than 2 drinks and to no more than 10 drinks spaced throughout a week. Pregnant women should not drink at all, because of possible damage to the fetus.

The evidence linking alcohol use with disease is strong. Excess alcohol increases the risk of liver damage, high blood pressure, and some forms of cancer. Like sugar, alcohol contains empty calories. Alcohol can kill the appetite for healthy food and affect how the body absorbs and uses nutrients in foods. Malnutrition is common in alcoholics. Protein and vitamin deficiencies can occur, resulting in anemia, neurological damage, and skin problems.

Even in moderate quantities, alcohol can affect balance, coordination, and judgment. Never drink before driving or operating machinery.

SPECIAL NUTRITIONAL ISSUES FOR WOMEN

Women have different nutritional needs at different ages and stages of their lives. Younger women need to replace iron loss from menstruation, while menopausal women must increase their calcium intake to compensate for the loss of the mineral that occurs during and after menopause. Pregnant and breast-feeding women need increased nutrients to nourish a growing baby. Understanding your nutritional needs allows you to avoid disease and be at your best throughout your life.

Menstruation

Women who are having monthly menstrual periods may need more iron in their diet, because they lose iron with the blood they shed each month. After women go through menopause, their RDAs for iron are the same as those for men. Meat, eggs, vegetables, and fortified cereals are good sources of iron. Some women may benefit from taking a daily multivitamin supplement that contains iron.

Before, During, and After Pregnancy

Pregnant women need to make certain changes in their diet to support both their own nutritional needs and that of the growing fetus. Making the correct nutritional changes before as well as after pregnancy can improve the health of mother and baby.

The Prepregnant Diet

A healthy diet in the period before conception is important. Carefully planned pregnancies allow women to make any necessary modifications to their diets before they become pregnant, ensuring that their babies will get the best possible start in life.

Many times a woman is pregnant for several weeks before she even suspects it. The first few weeks of fetal growth and development are critical; during this time, all the major organ systems are forming. Evidence is growing that birth defects affecting the spine and brain (neural tube defects) may be caused by a lack of folic acid in the earliest weeks of pregnancy. Some doctors recommend that women planning a pregnancy be sure to get enough folic acid from foods in their diet, or take a daily supplement of 0.4 milligrams. Folic acid is found in liver, leafy vegetables, oranges, peanuts, peas, beans, and lentils.

Pregnancy can strain your body's reserves of nutrients, especially iron and calcium. Build them up before pregnancy, if possible.

The Pregnancy Diet

Women who eat a well-balanced, healthy diet need to make only a few changes in their food intake during pregnancy. In particular, a moderate increase is needed in the number of calories and amount of iron, protein, folic acid, calcium, and phosphorus consumed.

It's not necessary to "eat for two," as the old adage says. Most pregnant women need about 300 calories per day extra to meet the needs of the growing baby. The exact amount depends on a recommended weight gain, which varies from woman to woman. If your weight was normal before you became pregnant, you should plan to gain 25 to 35 pounds. Underweight women can gain more—28 to 40 pounds—as can women carrying twins (35 to 45 pounds). Overweight women should gain less—about 15 to 25 pounds. Pregnancy is not the time to try to lose weight, either. Most of the extra nutrients needed can come from your regular diet (see Tables 3.1 and 3.4 for sources of these nutrients). To get the extra calories and nutrients, choose a moderately high number of servings from each of the food groups in the Food Guide Pyramid (See Fig. 1.1):

- Breads: 9 servings
- Vegetables: 4 servings
- Fruits: 3 servings
- Dairy products: 3 servings
- Meats: 3 servings

You may find it more comfortable to eat several small meals or snacks rather than eating three large meals.

For some nutrients, especially iron, it may be difficult to get all the needed amount from the diet alone. Your doctor may prescribe multivitamin supplements with iron. If you are a vegetarian, work with your doctor to plan a beneficial diet. If you eat milk and eggs, you may still be able to provide for all the baby's needs. Complete vegetarians, however, may need to take supplements.

Some women, especially African-Americans, have a condition called *lactose intolerance*, which means their bodies are unable to digest the sugar in milk products. Women who are lactose intolerant may need to limit their intake of dairy products to avoid possible gas and cramping. Instead, they should take a calcium supplement that provides about 1 gram of calcium per day.

In general, though, do not exceed the RDA for any nutrient, because some vitamins can be harmful if taken in excess. Too much vitamin A, for example, can cause birth defects.

As stated previously, avoid alcohol if you are pregnant. If you drink, you increase the risk that your child will be born with *fetal alcohol syndrome,* a condition that includes facial defects and varying degrees of mental retardation. The more you drink, the higher the risk. Because no one knows what constitutes a "safe" level of drinking during pregnancy, it's best not to drink alcohol at all.

Some women feel strong urges to eat nonfood items such as laundry starch or clay. This type of craving is called *pica.* If you experience this compulsion, discuss it with your doctor. Pica can be a sign of a nutritional deficiency, or it may cause deficiencies.

The Postpregnancy Diet

Once the baby is born, many women wonder how soon they can drop to their prepregnancy weight. Although women lose about 18 to 20 pounds within 10 days after birth, many women do end up weighing more than they did before. Weight gain is not absolute, however, if you begin a sensible weight loss plan right after birth. If you are not breast-feeding, choose low-fat options and keep to the low end of the recommended number of servings indicated by the Food Guide Pyramid. Include regular exercise in your fitness program.

If you are breast-feeding, you may need the same or even more nutrients than you did during pregnancy. Do not plan to lose much weight while you are breast-feeding. You can, however, lose a little weight slowly, perhaps 2 pounds a month, and still produce enough milk for your infant. (A nursing mother needs 500 to 600 more calories per day than she needed before she became pregnant.) Additional amounts of some nutrients are needed for breast-feeding (see Table 3.3), but these can usually be obtained from a well-balanced diet. Women who are lactose intolerant, vegetarians, or who cannot get the vitamins they need from their diet may need supplementation.

Generally, whatever you eat and drink is passed into your breast milk. Nutrients in the milk provide for the baby's growth and development. Harmful substances can end up in the milk as well, however. Alcohol can affect the baby if you have three or more drinks per day. Too much caffeine may also be harmful to your child. If you consume more than three cups of coffee (or the equivalent) per day, your breast-fed baby may be irritable and have trouble sleeping. Just about any medications you take can be found in your breast milk, too. If you are taking medication, check with your doctor before you begin breast-feeding your baby.

Menopause

By the time a woman reaches her early 50s, her periods become erratic and gradually end. For women in the United States, the average age at the last menstrual period is about 51 years. Women who have had their ovaries removed by surgery go through an immediate menopause, called a surgical menopause.

After menopause, a woman no longer produces as much of the female hormone estrogen. Estrogen provides some protection against heart disease. Once estrogen production slows down, it is especially important to eat a diet low in fat, saturated fat and cholesterol.

The loss of estrogen also affects the bones. Around and after menopause, the rate of bone loss increases, and may cause a condition called *osteoporosis*. If too much calcium and protein are lost, bones can become spongy and brittle. Risk factors for osteoporosis include being thin and being white or Asian. Smoking and a sedentary lifestyle or excessive exercise also increase your risk for bone loss. Many doctors recommend that postmenopausal women get 1,500 milligrams of calcium each day. The main sources of calcium in the diet are dairy products, but calcium is also found in green leafy vegetables, tofu (bean curd), and fish with bones. Women who are lactose intolerant or who are vegetarians may be able to get enough calcium from nondairy sources. For some, supplements are a good idea. Avoid eating too much protein, which can even be harmful because it causes the body to flush out needed calcium. Also minimize drinking carbonated soft drinks that are high in phosphorus (which flushes calcium from the system) and limit caffeine. You need enough vitamins to keep the minerals in the bones.

Exercise during the postmenopausal years is still vital. It helps burn fat and strengthens the heart. It also strengthens bones, which protects against osteoporosis, and strengthens muscles, which improves balance and prevents falls.

THE LATER YEARS

Women who are 65 years or older have special dietary needs of their own. For one, older women need fewer daily calories than younger women, because the body's metabolism tends to slow down as people age. Older women also tend to be less active than younger women. The foods that provide the calories needed to maintain a healthy weight may not be enough to provide enough nutrients, so a multivitamin supplement is a good idea.

Osteoporosis continues to be a major health risk for older women. Approximately 33 percent of women over age 65 will suffer a fracture of the spine, and by age 90, 33 percent of all women will have experienced a hip fracture. Older women should be sure to get enough calcium in their diets, keep up with moderate exercise, and be careful to avoid falls.

Although good nutrition is key for an older woman's health, changes in the body present special dietary challenges. The senses of taste and smell may decline so that foods seem less appetizing, for example. Different seasonings may need to be used, but it is a good idea to try herbs and spices rather than just adding more salt. If older women have lost some teeth or have poor-fitting dentures, they may find it difficult to eat. Careful attention should be paid to dental care and proper denture fit.

Loss of appetite may be a problem in the very elderly, causing malnutrition. In severe cases, food supplements or feeding through a tube may be necessary. Older women may not be outside enough to produce adequate amounts of vitamin D, so they may need supplements of this vitamin, too.

VEGETARIANS

Women may adopt a vegetarian diet for reasons of religion, moral beliefs, or health. Those who eat dairy products and eggs in addition to plant foods are called *lacto-ovo vegetarians.* Those who eat foods only of plant origin are called *vegans,* or *complete vegetarians.*

If you are a vegetarian, choose your foods carefully to be sure that you get all the essential amino acids (the protein building blocks that your body does not manufacture) from your diet. If you eat a variety of foods daily all the needed amino acids will likely be provided. For example, beans or peas can be combined with rice; grains plus legumes and nuts plus seeds are other good combinations. Because soy protein has the best amino acid makeup of the vegetable protein sources, use products made from soy, such as tofu.

Vegetarians should be especially alert to the presence of iron, calcium, and vitamin B_{12} in their diets. Beans, seeds, nuts, green leafy vegetables, dried fruits, and grains are good sources of iron, as are fortified cereals. Calcium can be found in green leafy vegetables and tofu in addition to dairy products. Because vitamin B_{12} is found naturally only in foods from animals, you may wish to eat more fortified breads and cereals or, better, take a daily supplement.

PART 2
Exercise and Physical Fitness

Janet Emily Freedman, M.D.

I t's official: Regular exercise can help women live longer, healthier lives. In the fall of 1992, the American Heart Association formally designated inactivity as one of the top four risk factors for the development of heart attack and stroke—the nation's number-one killer of women every year. Along with high blood pressure, cigarette smoking, and high cholesterol, the lack of exercise is a contributing factor in cardiovascular disease.

Women and exercise did not always go together. Historically, women were not encouraged to go "all out" physically. Certainly it was viewed as unfeminine for women to actually sweat. Fortunately, we have come a long way in just about every sport and physical activity you can name.

Due in part to Title IX of the Educational Assistance Act (which requires all educational institutions receiving federal monies to offer equal opportunities to women and girls to train and compete in sports) more and more women have entered professional sports in the past few decades. In 1970, two years before Title IX, no woman had ever finished in the New York City Marathon. In 1994, the top woman finisher ran the course in 2 hours, 27 minutes—just 16 minutes behind the male finisher. In recent Olympic games, American women have brought home more medals than their male colleagues.

Most women have neither the time, the training, nor the desire to compete in sports on the level of the highly trained "elite" athlete, but we can all enjoy the proven benefits of an exercise program.

WHAT EXERCISE CAN DO FOR YOU

The Health Connection

The news is easy medicine to swallow: Exercise prevents disease. By exercising regularly, you can significantly lower your risk of a myriad of diseases that are influenced by obesity and inactivity.

Exercise appears to help prevent cardiovascular disease, including heart attacks, stroke, and high blood pressure, by lowering low-density lipoproteins (the so-called "bad" cholesterol), increasing high-density lipoproteins (the "good" cholesterol), and lowering resting blood pressure and heart rate. There is some evidence that consistent exercise may be related to decreased rates of certain cancers, specifically breast and ovarian cancer, but strong scientific evidence is not yet available.

One of the most widespread diseases in the United States, diabetes mellitus, is also affected by physical inactivity. Recent studies show that regular exercise cuts in half the risk of developing adult-onset diabetes; burning just 500 extra calories a week decreases the risk of developing the disease by as much as 6 percent.

The Emotional Connection

Exercise has been called nature's tranquilizer because it has been shown to break up stress patterns

BENEFITS OF REGULAR EXERCISE

- promotes weight loss and decreased body fat
- decreases risk of cardiovascular disease
- lowers blood pressure
- decreases insulin use in diabetics
- prevents osteoporosis
- lowers serum cholesterol
- raises serum HDL
- slows aging of heart and lungs
- slows age-related muscle loss
- reduces back pain
- improves self-image

Possible Benefits of Exercise

- lowers rates of breast cancer
- lowers rates of ovarian cancer
- lessens labor pain
- lessens menstrual cramps/PMS
- strengthens immune system

in the body. Exercise affects the brain and the emotions in many complex ways. Many exercisers report feeling good after a workout. This is due to the release during vigorous exercise of body chemicals called endorphins, which are known to dull pain and produce a mild euphoria.

Exercise and Weight Control

Exercise and weight control are often linked together, and it's easy to see why. Your body weight is the result of a complex interaction between the food you consume, your physical activity, and your body's metabolism. Exercise alone, or exercise in combination with a sensible diet, can help you lose weight and keep it off. Exercise can also help you maintain your ideal weight even as your metabolism slows down as you age. (After the age of 35, it takes fewer calories and more exercise to avoid putting on weight.) Women who are only 10 percent above their ideal weight may be able to achieve weight loss with exercise alone. Twenty minutes of vigorous exercise can burn up as much as 300 calories per session.
Exercise promotes weight loss in several ways.

■ *Exercise increases your metabolic rate.* Between the ages of 20 and 50, about 70 percent of your body's energy expenditure is to maintain the resting metabolic rate—the sum of all processes or chemical reactions in the body, such as digesting food and maintaining body temperature. Thirty percent is used for physical exertion. Exercise not only increases energy use for physical exertion, but also causes an increase in the resting metabolic rate, which may last as long as 48 hours after exercise. A regular exercise pro-

WHY DIETS DON'T WORK

Most weight-loss plans are poorly designed and don't result in permanent weight loss. In fact, diets based on limiting your caloric intake for a certain period of time—especially fad diets and crash diets—are doomed to failure. You may lose a few pounds by starving yourself, but as soon as you stop the dieting, your body will return to its previous weight. Even worse, repeated weight loss and weight gain from dieting—called the "yo-yo syndrome"—makes it harder to lose weight the next time around and may be dangerous to your general health.

The only recommended way to lose weight and to keep it off is to change your eating habits permanently (behavior modification) and increase your physical activity on a regular basis (exercise).

gram burns calories, therefore, even on your "off" days.

In addition, the single biggest factor in producing a higher resting metabolic rate is the amount of your lean body, or muscle, tissue. Muscle tissue is highly active, even when at rest, eating up a great deal of energy to sustain itself. On average, it accounts for five times as much of our total daily energy expenditure as fat. So the more total muscle you have, the higher your metabolism and the less fat you accumulate.

- *Exercise preserves muscle.* Dieting alone causes loss of body fat and muscle mass equally. Exercising *plus* eating a nutritious low-fat diet shifts the balance toward reducing fat and keeping muscle—the desired effect. This important shift occurs because active muscle tissue burns more fat for its energy needs and because the fibers are using the available food supply more efficiently.

- *Exercise may be an appetite suppressant.* Many women who exercise believe they eat less and feel less hungry. It has been suggested that if you exercise about two hours before a meal, you may actually eat less. It has not been proven that exercising actually diminishes your appetite—perhaps you eat less because you are "revved up" and feeling good. Research also suggests that mild exercise *after* meals may also help in controlling weight gain. A light exercise, such as walking, allows digestion to continue and can aid in the movement of food through the digestive tract.

TYPES OF EXERCISE

There are two basic types of exercise: aerobic and anaerobic.

Aerobic exercise improves cardiovascular health by forcing the body to deliver larger amounts of oxygen to working muscles. (The word *aerobic* is derived from a Greek word meaning "air.") With regular aerobic exercise, your heart increases its ability to pump blood and deliver oxygen to your body's tissues efficiently. In addition, your muscles will develop a greater capacity to use this oxygen and your heart will become stronger. It also allows your heart to rest longer between beats even when exercising.

Anaerobic exercise, or exercise "without air," strengthens individual muscles that draw on their own sources of energy and do not require the body to increase its supply of oxygen. Anaerobic exercise, which includes muscle conditioning or weight training, builds muscle mass while keeping the body strong and flexible.

Since a major health concern among women is the threat of osteoporosis (loss of bone mass), it is important to add another term to the physical fitness lexicon: *weight-bearing exercise.* These exercises provide the stress of muscles contracting or pulling on bones, in effect adding to the force of gravity. Exercises such as walking, running, aerobic dancing, and weight training all help to maintain or build bone mass.

THE EXERCISE PRESCRIPTION: TRAINING

The benefits of exercise come as the result of training, which means adapting the body to exercise over time. It is important to note that when it comes to exercise, men and women are not created equally. We must train longer and harder to achieve equal capacity for prolonged exercise.

Women should train to improve in several areas:

- *Strength.* Strength is the ability of a muscle to apply or resist a force. It determines how much weight a weightlifter can lift at any one time, or how steep a hill a bicyclist can pedal. Because women produce little of the male hormone testosterone, we have less strength than men with the same body weight. We also have a higher percentage of body fat, so we have pro-portionally less muscle. Our muscles do respond well to strength training, however, so strength training should be a part of your exer-cise program. You can develop strength and muscle tone by practicing repeated muscle con-tractions against resistance.

- *Endurance.* Endurance is the ability to repeat an activity over an extended period of time—to bike or run longer distances or lift a weight repeatedly. Surprisingly, women have a greater ability to train for endurance than do men. This phenomenon is not clearly understood, but many exercise experts believe that once all barriers to equality in training disappear, women will surpass men in some endurance activities.

- *Flexibility.* Flexibility is the ability of the mus-cles, tendons, and ligaments to move easily at the joints. Women are more flexible in this area than men, whose larger muscles can inhibit movement of joints. This ability may be hor-monally related—we know, for example, that flexibility increases during pregnancy. Also, flex-ibility is not tied to strength—witness some weight lifters who have difficulty touching their toes.

- *Aerobic capacity.* This refers to the ability of the heart and lungs to deliver oxygen to the muscles, and the ability of the muscles to use that oxygen efficiently. Women have smaller hearts and lungs and generally begin training with less aerobic capacity than do men of similar size. Your aerobic capacity can be improved by increasing the heart rate through steady, sustained exercise for at least 20 minutes three times per week. It is not necessary to do exercises faster but rather to do them over a longer period. The heart becomes stronger and more efficient; it beats more slowly, but each beat pumps more blood. The lungs become larger and stronger, moving more oxygen in and more carbon dioxide out.

HOW TO PLAN A GOOD EXERCISE PROGRAM

To achieve a healthy balance, it is important to maintain a balance between too much and too little exercise. Not exercising frequently enough will greatly lengthen the time needed to achieve the beneficial effects of exercise. On the other hand, workouts need not be complicated or exhausting to be effective. The truth is that more is not always better when it comes to exercise (see box below). Beginners in particular may err on the side of overdoing it, perhaps trying to make up for lost time. And exercising too frequently will not improve aerobic capacity, strength, or endurance any faster and may, in fact, lead to more frequent injuries. Working too hard can also cause fatigue and muscle cramping.

If you wish to exercise daily, alternate types of activity between an aerobic day and a stretching or weight training day. Or alternate swimming, which is almost injury-proof, with some other aerobic activity. (If you use weights, it is recommended that you lift no more than two or three times a week, because muscle fibers need 48 hours to recover.) You need one day every week without vigorous exercise so that your body can rest and recover. You can walk on an "off" day, but don't run.

Conventional wisdom used to be to check with a physician before starting any exercise program, but it is now believed that the benefits of pre-exercise examinations have been overstated. Generally it is not necessary to get a doctor's approval if you are in good health, unless you are over 35 and sedentary or in a risk category because you are a heavy smoker, overweight, or have diabetes, hypertension, or high cholesterol. Your doctor may then recommend an exercise cardiogram, which measures heart electrical function, but even that test is sometimes misleading as it rarely detects abnormalities in women who have no obvious symptoms of heart disease.

Sample Workout

1. *Warm-up.* Warming up is an essential part of any exercise program, regardless of the level of difficulty. It is as important to warm up before a brisk

walk as before a marathon. At rest, the large muscles of the body have very little blood flow, and a sudden increase in the demand on these muscles requires an increase in blood and oxygen. Similarly, muscles, tendons, and ligaments are at their shortest length while at rest, and exercise can suddenly stretch them, causing injuries.

Warming up consists of gentle stretching of the body parts that will be exercised, followed by a *gradual* increase in activity. Runners, for example, should warm up with stretches for the legs (Figure 2.1), then do some walking or slow running; bicyclists may warm up with walking or pedaling slowly on a level surface. Most exercisers develop their own warm-up routine, which should be longer on cold days. (It is also a healthy idea to dress in layers that can be taken off during warm-up.)

Pay particular attention to certain areas of the body that may be abused over the normal course of a day. For example, wearing high heels may cause shortened Achilles tendons, and sedentary desk jobs can also result in shortened hamstring muscles. If you do keyboard work, you may experience shortness and tension in the muscles of the neck. You need to lengthen these muscles during warm-up and stretching. Some simple rules:

- Stretch until tension is felt. The feeling should be tightness or mild burning, but never pain. Hold for 10 to 20 seconds. (Figure 2.2.)

- Do not bounce; stretch out like a cat. Bouncing can cause tears in muscles and can lead to scars, calcium deposits, and ultimately, decreased flexibility.

■ Stretch every day, at least to start. After several months, flexibility can be maintained with stretching every other day. (Some women choose to incorporate yoga into their routines. Yoga strengthens, stretches, and relaxes the body.)

2. *Aerobic Exercise.* The bulk of your exercise program should be devoted to an aerobic workout. The eventual goal is 20 to 30 minutes of aerobic exercise that increases the heart rate. Beginners should exercise aerobically only 5 to 10 minutes, building up their endurance over six or more weeks. Running, stair climbing, cross-country skiing, bicycling, rowing, aerobic dance, and brisk walking all are good workout choices.

In order for aerobic exercise to have a healthy effect, it must be of sufficient intensity. Exercise at your target heart rate (see box on "Target Heart Rate").

3. *Muscle Conditioning.* Although a level of physical fitness can be maintained with aerobic conditioning alone, many women find the benefits of weight training to be well worth the extra time and effort. A weight-training and muscle-conditioning routine involves about 30 minutes of slow but constant stress on different muscles of the body. An adequate weight-lifting routine can be formulated with an exercise specialist in a gym, but generally speaking it should consist of about a dozen exercises: six for the upper body and six for the lower.

4. *Cool-down.* When you finish exercising, it is crucial to have at least 5 to 10 minutes of slowly decreasing activity followed by stretching so that your heart rate, breathing, and body temperature can

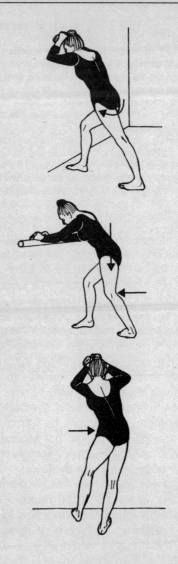

Figure 2.1. Stretching out before any type of exercise can help prevent injuries. Here are some general guidelines:

• *Never stretch a cold muscle.* Do some brisk walking or jogging slowly in place to warm up your muscles before stretching them.

• *Don't bounce.* Hold the stretch to a count of 30, release, and then repeat. Bouncing during the stretch can cause muscle injury.

• *Don't forget to breathe!* Breathe in deeply and then exhale slowly as you go into the stretch. Don't tense up—relax into the stretch, breathing deeply, slowly and regularly.

Top: Calf stretch. To stretch the gastrocnemius (calf) muscle, stand facing a wall with your right knee bent and your left leg stretched out straight behind you. Push in toward the wall, keeping your back straight, your left leg straight, and your heel flat on the floor. You should feel the stretching sensation in the back of your calf and knee. To prevent injury during this stretch, do not let your right knee extend forward past your toes. Repeat with the other leg.

Middle: Soleus stretch. The soleus muscle lies underneath the gastrocnemius. To stretch it, bring your left leg in toward the wall, bending your left knee and keeping your heel flat on the floor, and press your left leg down into the floor. This stretch is a little harder to get right than the calf stretch; practice adjusting your position until you feel the stretch deep in your calf muscle. Like the calf stretch, the soleus stretch should not cause your right knee to extend forward past your toes. Repeat with the other leg.

Bottom: Hip stretch. To stretch the muscles that surround the hip, lean your upper body against a wall with your weight on your right leg. Place your left leg slightly forward with the knee bent, and push toward the right with your hips. Repeat on the other side.

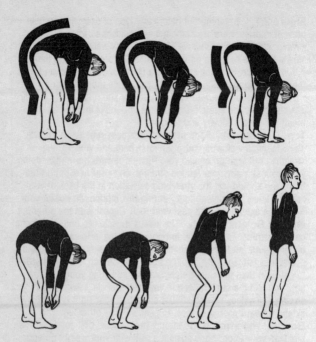

Figure 2.2. Lower-Body Stretch. Stretching out your back, hips, groin area, and thigh muscles is a good idea before any type of exercise.

Top: This stretch will loosen your hamstrings, the group of muscles in the backs of your thighs. From a standing position, slowly bend forward and over as far as comfortably possible. Don't lock your knees—allow them to bend naturally. If you can, continue the stretch until you touch your toes, and then place your hands flat on the floor. Do not force this stretch, or you may pull a muscle in the back of your leg. Hold for 30 seconds and release; as with all stretches, do not bounce.

Bottom: After holding the stretch, slowly rise to a standing position with your head down and arms hanging forward. Think of your spine as "uncurling," and feel the stretch work up your back.

YOUR TARGET HEART RATE

Your maximum heart rate is calculated by subtracting your age from 220. As you exercise, try to achieve your *target heart rate,* which is 60 to 80 percent of your maximum heart rate. (Figure 2.3.)

TRAINING HEART RATES BY AGE

Age	60%	80%
30	114	152
35	111	148
40	108	144
45	105	140
50	102	136
55	99	132
60	96	128

For example, if you are an average 50-year-old, your maximum heart rate is 220 minus 50, or 170. Your target heart rate is from 102 to 136 beats per minute, 60 to 80 percent of your maximum heart rate.

return to rest levels. In a proper cool-down, more blood is delivered to the skin, which helps eliminate heat and literally cools you off. Cooling down also helps the body rid the muscles of waste products—chemicals produced by the muscles during exercise—that are in part responsible for the achy "charley horse" feeling the day after strenuous exercise.

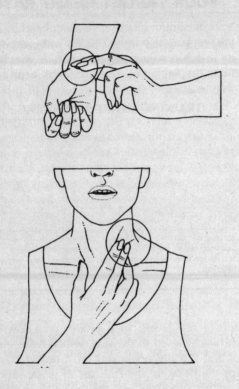

Figure 2.3. Taking your pulse can be done most easily by feeling it on the inside of your wrist (top) or in the carotid artery in the side of your neck (bottom). Press lightly with two fingers on one of these two pulse points; you may need to move your fingers around a little to find your pulse. Once you do, count the beats you feel for six seconds, then multiply by 10 to get the number of beats per minute; this is your heart rate.

HOW TO PREVENT INJURY

Two decades ago, women athletes suffered injuries at rates far higher than those of male athletes. This dismal record led to the incorrect conclusion that women were more prone to injury and unable to participate in sports at the same level as men. The truth is that women were (and sometimes still are) denied the thorough training afforded male athletes and that successful training techniques used by men are not always directly applicable to women. With proper training, women athletes' injury rates are dropping to a level roughly equivalent to that of men.

But, no matter what exercise you choose, no exercise is injury-proof. Name a body part and there is probably a sports-related concern, from swimmer's ear to tennis elbow. Blisters, bumps, and strains are common to most sports. Different types of activities also stress different parts of the body. For example, running stresses the lower leg, bicycling taxes the upper leg, and tennis and squash involve sudden stops that can hurt the knee, ankle, and lower back.

Some exercises are safer than others. For example, swimming (despite some ear problems) is generally considered a safe exercise for just about everyone—even the disabled. Similarly, brisk walking can be undertaken by almost any able-bodied woman. Jogging, on the other hand, puts pressure on weight-bearing body parts and can be particularly unsafe if you run regularly on hard surfaces such as concrete or asphalt.

Exercise-related injuries are of two kinds: *acute*

injury, which occurs suddenly as the result of a single accident or misuse (such as a twist or fall), and *overuse* injury, which occurs as the result of an activity that is constantly repeated and strains the body over a long period of time. A proper exercise program should include injury prevention activities. Several elements are involved.

For one, exercise and physical activity should *never* be painful. Don't accept the oft-repeated saw "No pain, no gain." Any pain experienced during or after exercise deserves investigation and should be eliminated. Such pain is usually due to improper mechanics or, more commonly, to overuse of muscles not yet strong enough for internal activity. The solution is to slow down the rate of progression of the exercise program. Also spot-strengthen specific muscles to help them catch up with the demands of the exercise.

Consider consulting an athletic trainer for advice on injury prevention and for help in designing a healthy fitness program. The trainer should have a degree in physical education and experience in prescribing exercise workouts for all types of students.

As previously discussed, warm-up and cooldown are absolutely essential to injury-free workouts. They may seem to be boring and unproductive parts of exercise, but if you are cool, stiff, or out of shape you can tear a ligament or tendon if you skip warmup. If you eliminate cool-down, the abrupt shift after strenuous exercise can cause fainting or worse. When first beginning an exercise program, the warm-up and cool-down periods should nearly equal the actual vigorous exercise in duration. As you get in shape and become better trained, these segments can drop in duration but should never be less than 10 to 15 minutes.

Be careful not to push yourself too fast and too far when first beginning an exercise program. Do half of what you think you can for at least three exercise sessions. This gives you the opportunity to test for areas of weakness and pain before overuse sets in. View increasing the level of exercise as a process that will take months, not weeks.

It is also important that you do not exercise if you have a fever or a viral infection. A mild workout will not make a cold worse, but exercising tends to raise body temperature and you don't want to exercise if you are already feeling hot. It is a myth that exercise "flushes" out illness, and overdoing it may be harmful to your muscles and heart.

Dehydration is a common cause of fatigue during workouts. As a rule, drink water before each workout and then drink several gulps of water every 10 to 15 minutes during the workout. The rule of thumb is: If you feel thirsty, it's too late—you're dehydrated.

Although exercise has an accumulated positive effect, unfortunately it can't be stored up to be used later. If you miss more than three consecutive exercise sessions, you will need to decrease the amount of exercise you have been doing and build up again. Your body loses improvement from exercise at a rate of between 5 and 10 percent per week of rest, and completely stopping exercise for one month results in a 50 percent decline. If you know in advance you have to reduce your exercise program, try to decrease the time spent during each session rather than decreasing the frequency—this will better preserve your gains.

To treat injuries, the general advice is RICE: *r*est (stop the activity); *i*ce (apply cold, which constricts blood vessels and limits swelling); *c*ompress (wrap a towel or cloth around the injury part); and *e*levate (raise the injury above the level of your heart). Do not immediately put heat on a wound. It increases blood flow, which causes swelling—but after 24 hours you can apply moist heat on a tear or sprain.

Several parts of a woman's body are highly susceptible to injury due to overuse, improper training, inadequate warm-up, poor flexibility, or inadequate equipment.

Knee Injuries

Knee injuries are especially common. The knee is a complex joint that undergoes tremendous stress during activities requiring repetitive bending (flexing) and straightening (extending) or a constantly flexed knee (such as volleyball, racquet sports, and downhill hiking). The major stabilizers are the quadriceps and hamstrings, the large muscles of the thigh. If very strong, these muscles can protect the knee joint from injury. Unfortunately, in many women these muscles are not strong enough, and knee pain and injury result.

When you seek a physician's opinion about knee pain, the knee should be thoroughly examined and a complete history of the pain taken, including the type and location of pain, aggravating activities, swelling, locking, and heat sensations. X-rays may or may not be indicated. You should be examined sitting and standing, with legs and feet completely undressed.

The *patella,* or kneecap, is a common site of knee pain. The patella is a small oval bone embedded in the tendons of the quadriceps muscle, and it rides over the knee joint as the knee bends and straightens. The line of movement of the patella is unique in each woman and is determined by the angle formed between the *tibia* bone of the lower leg, the *femur* in the thigh, and the strength of the quadriceps muscle. This line of movement is called the *Q angle.* The Q angle is larger in women than in men and if very large may result in abnormal patellar movement and pain.

Chondromalacia

Chondromalacia is a condition in which the cartilage on the undersurface of the patella is degenerating. In the early stages of the condition, the cartilage swells and softens, and cracks form on the surface. Pain increases when the knee flexes beyond 90 degrees, and the sufferer will find going downstairs more painful than going up. Extending the knee generally decreases the pain. On physical examination, there may be pain on the underside of the edge of the patella. Abnormal movement of the patella may or may not be seen.

The degeneration of the cartilage and the pain of chondromalacia is not a disease in itself but a response to abnormal or excessive forces on the knee. In virtually all but the most severe cases, the most important treatment is strengthening of the quadriceps and hamstring muscles. Surgery is generally not recommended until a complete trial of exercises has been completed.

Achilles Tendinitis

Achilles tendinitis is injury to or inflammation of the Achilles tendon, also called the heel cord, located in the back of the ankle. Achilles tendinitis is common in running and jumping activities. Women who have been wearing high-heeled shoes for many years may have shortened Achilles tendons and may be prone to developing tendinitis. The pain is located at the top of the back of the heel and increases with ankle movement. It may be worse in the morning.

Treatment includes rest and, if severe, crutches and a cast or ankle splint. Local heat or ice and anti-inflammatory medication are helpful. In the acute phase, a heel lift will shorten the tendon and relieve pain. Once pain is reduced, gentle stretching is started to return the tendon to normal length (Figure 2.4). Prevention of Achilles tendinitis includes avoiding high heels and thorough stretching of the Achilles tendon prior to exercise.

Shin Splints

Shin splints are the occurrence of pain along the front and middle of the lower leg, felt during or after running, walking, or hiking. Shin splints are caused by many tiny tears in the muscles attaching to the tibia, the large bone of the lower leg. The problem is caused by the impact of the foot on the ground and is

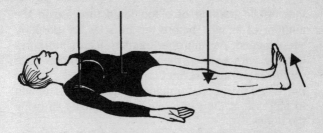

Figure 2.4.   Foot Stretches. Gently stretching an injured Achilles tendon—after swelling and pain have been reduced—can help return it to normal length. Lie flat on your back with your shoulders, hips, and knees touching the floor and your legs straight. Slowly bring your toes up toward you as far as you can without pain.

worsened by running on a hard surface, wearing worn or insufficiently padded shoes, weak leg muscles, and insufficient warm-up stretching. Treatment includes rest, local heat and/or ice, well-padded shoes, and proper stretching (Figure 2.5). Persistent shin splint pain that does not go away quickly should be evaluated by a doctor.

Stress Fractures

Stress fractures are far more common in women than in men. The most common sites for stress fractures are the bones of the foot and leg. In older women who have experienced menopause, stress fractures may be due to the bone weakness that results from osteoporosis. Except in highly trained athletes, stress fractures in young exercising women are the result of incomplete training or a too rapid increase in the amount of activity before the muscles are properly strengthened. As improper training occurs more frequently with women than with men, women have greater rates of stress fracture. Stress fractures can be prevented by gradual training to allow bone strength to increase at the same rate as the activity stressing the bones.

The pain of a stress fracture is generally limited to the area of the broken bone and increases with continued activity. There may not be swelling, and X-rays may not show the fracture until 2–3 weeks after injury. Treatment involves rest. A cast is generally not required, although crutches or a cane may be. Recovery and return to activity should involve a muscle strengthening program.

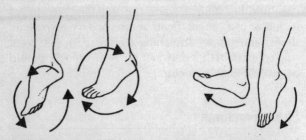

Figure 2.5. Treatment for shin splints includes stretching the tibialis anterior (shin) muscle in the front of the lower leg. These stretches can be done while sitting or lying down.
Top: Raise your toes as far up toward your upper body as possible; hold, then stretch them downward as far as they will go.
Bottom: Rotate your ankle in either direction, making a circle as large as possible. Repeat in the other direction.

STICKING WITH YOUR EXERCISE PLAN

Beginning an exercise program is easy; maintaining it is the difficult part. Women who smoke, are overweight, have little free time, or begin an overambitious program are at highest risk of dropping out. To improve your chances of maintaining your exercise program, keep these tips in mind:

- Any exercise is better than none. Although aerobic training requires at least 15–20 minutes three times per week, any vigorous exercise burns calories and increases circulation, flexibility, and endurance.

- To avoid boredom, select an activity that is suited to your personality. Exercise can be social (aerobic class, running with a partner, hiking trips) or solitary (jogging, swimming, stair climbing). Increasingly women are exercising their competitive side by joining teams. There are now women's leagues in just about every sport, including basketball, softball, bowling, and karate.

- Set reasonable goals. A program that is too strenuous is at best discouraging and painful; at worst, it may cause injury. Start slowly and build gradually; expect the first stages to be awkward, boring, and even frustrating.

- Do not expect noticeable gains for at least 4 to 6 weeks. The good news is that unfit people enjoy fast initial improvement: unused muscles and tissues react swiftly to regular workouts. But increasing muscle strength and endurance requires actual changes in the muscle tissue, which takes time.

- Do not begin exercising with a male partner. Even an out-of-shape man has greater strength and endurance than an out-of-shape woman of the same age, size, and general health. A man will be able to do more and advance faster than you will, which may frustrate you. If you want to exercise with someone, choose a partner of the same sex, age, and ability.

- If you are significantly overweight, try not to set yourself up for almost certain failure. It makes sense, for example, not to join a gym that caters to primarily fit, thin women. Begin instead by walking or working out with another overweight buddy.

- Put your best foot forward, literally, by buying well-fitting athletic shoes. Highly specialized shoes—for tennis, walking, or basketball—are popular but are often unnecessary and costly. Make sure whatever shoe you choose is cushioned, gives you enough toe room, and has a padded insole and good arch support. If you exercise regularly, have a pair of shoes devoted only to exercise and allow them to dry completely before each use.

- Do not spend a fortune on unnecessary or inappropriate clothing. Wear clothing that is comfortable and loose, such as sweats. Fabrics should be stretchy, absorbent, and made of natural fibers or fiber blends. One-hundred-percent artificial fibers can, in fact, increase your risk of dehydration.

- Similarly, do not spend a great deal of money on exercise machines and specialized equipment. Most home exercise equipment sits collecting dust or winds up in your next tag sale. If possible, try out any equipment you are considering buying at your local gym. (You can test an exercise tape by renting it first from your local video store.) Be particularly wary of equipment advertised on television that claims to help firm specific parts of your body. This equipment is often no better than a general exercise program, and some of the items may actually increase your risk of injury. Watch out for any exaggerated claims ("Lose eight inches overnight without breaking a sweat!"); there is no substitute for physical activity.

EXERCISE AND MENSTRUATION

Menstruation itself does not affect athletic performance. World records and Olympic medals have been won by women in all phases of their menstrual cycle. In fact, exercise tends to ease cramps, and many women athletes experience less pain at that time. Unless you suffer from excessive bleeding, you can exercise as hard as you like during menstruation.

Severe changes in the menstrual cycle occur rarely, and only among women who are training at collegiate or Olympic levels. Certain sports have been more closely associated with disruption of the menstrual cycle—running, gymnastics, and figure skating. Although the cause of menstrual cycle changes in athletes is not well understood, it is believed to be due to a combination of an extreme amount of exercise, increased lean body mass, inadequate nutrition, and competition-related stress.

Menstrual changes include amenorrhea (no periods); oligomenorrhea (light periods); cycles without ovulation; and delayed menarche (late age of onset). Exercise-induced menstrual dysfunction generally resolves once training decreases. There are, however, long-term consequences to prolonged exercise-related menstrual cycle disruption. Amenorrheic athletes suffer bone loss at a rate similar to that of women in menopause, and they may have a greater risk of fractures later in life.

It must be stressed that these potentially serious consequences are experienced by a very small number of highly trained athletes. The average exercising woman experiences no menstrual changes and, as noted, usually benefits greatly from exercise. Do not assume that menstrual irregularities are caused by exercise. If you are exercising and experience menstrual changes, consult your physician. In addition, any vaginal bleeding that occurs between menstrual periods, no matter how strenuous the workout, is abnormal and should also be discussed with your physician.

EXERCISE AND YOUR BREASTS

Some women are concerned—in part due to some misconceptions—about the effect strenuous exercise can have on their breasts.

There is no evidence that contact sports result in any serious breast trauma. If anything, the fatty parts of the breast protect the other parts from becoming injured. When trauma to the breast does occur, it does not cause anything more than a bruise, which rarely requires any treatment. It does not lead to the development of breast cancer, cause difficulty in breast feeding, or promote any other breast disease or condition. Women with breast implants, however, should avoid contact sports, as trauma may cause rupture of the implant or bleeding of breast tissue.

The nipples are more vulnerable, however. "Runner's nipples" is a condition of abrasion and irritation of the nipples caused by the rubbing off of the outer layer of the skin as the exerciser runs or bounces during exercise. You can prevent this condition by wearing a supportive bra without seams, putting Band-Aids or nursing pads over the nipples during exercise, and wearing warm outer clothing in cold weather. You can also give the nipples a chance to heal by switching exercise activities, using a different type of movement on alternative days.

There is no evidence that exercise either enlarges or reduces the actual size of your breasts. Because the breast consists of predominantly fatty tissue, loss of overall body fat leads to some fat loss from the breasts as well.

The myth persists that exercise involving bouncing will cause the breast to sag. This is not true. This misconception may be based on the fact that the connective tissue that attaches the breast to the body does not seem to offer structural support. Sagging, when it does occur, is a result of breast size, weight, and age. It *is* a fact, though, that large-breasted women may find physical activity uncomfortable unless their breasts are supported by a well-fitting sports bra. Sports bras should be snug and strong enough to hold you and keep you from bouncing but light enough to breathe. Avoid bras that ride up or have bones or wires.

EXERCISE AND PREGNANCY

In the past, the ideal activity during pregnancy was rest or "confinement." The general consensus today is that most activities can be safely continued during and after pregnancy. Even women who have never exercised before can begin a limited exercise program when they are pregnant.

The health benefits of mild to moderate exercise are generally positive for the mother. Active women gain less weight and have less subjective distress during labor, although the length of labor is unchanged.

You need to make some concessions to your burgeoning size, however. For example, there are changes in the cardiopulmonary system: the heart

WHO SHOULD NOT EXERCISE DURING PREGNANCY

The American College of Obstetricians and Gynecologists suggests the following as contraindications to vigorous exercise during pregnancy:

- any heart or lung disease;
- history or risk of premature labor;
- history of three or more miscarriages;
- incompetent cervix;
- multiple gestation (twins, etc.);
- ruptured membrane.

In addition, consult a doctor before starting an exercise program if you are hypertensive, overweight, or extremely sedentary.

rate is faster, the volume of blood larger, and the stroke volume (the amount of blood pumped per beat) increased. The growing fetus puts an additional demand on your energy. It is as if the body is already performing mild exercise, so there is less reserve left for additional exertion. You will also be more easily fatigued and find you have a decreased exercise tolerance.

In the beginning of your pregnancy, you can continue your pre-pregnancy exercise program with only a few modifications. All exercise should include warm-up and cool-down periods to prevent injury to lax joints: muscles stretch, ligaments soften, and joints loosen to make room for the baby. Stretching and strengthening (particularly of the abdominal muscles) and weight training are acceptable for uncomplicated pregnancies (Figure 2.6). Exercise performed in the supine position (lying on the back) should be limited by the second trimester. This position not only causes back pain, but also results in the uterus compressing the large blood vessels and decreases blood flow to the uterus. Similarly, the Valsalva maneuver (increasing abdominal pressure while holding the breath) decreases blood flow to the uterus and should be avoided. Activities which may result in Valsalva include weightlifting and rowing.

Walking and swimming can continue throughout pregnancy and are excellent choices if you are just beginning to exercise: They build endurance, strengthen muscles, and improve circulation and respiration. Avoid activities such as fencing. Jogging, volleyball, and tennis—activities that involve impact and balance—need to be reduced and stopped altogether by the third trimester. Bicycle riding and cross-country skiing should also be tapered off by the third trimester.

Some guidelines for exercising during pregnancy are based on the knowledge that hyperthermia (high body temperature) can be dangerous to both mother and fetus. We know that exercise, in general, raises body temperature; sustained strenuous aerobic activity can increase maternal body temperature, often to as high as 102° F. To be safe, then, it is advised you check your temperature at the end of each exercise session. If it exceeds 101° F, take immediate steps to stay cool. To further prevent hyperthermia and reduce the risk of injury due to fatigue, a limit of 15 minutes of exercise at maximum level of exertion (see box on "Your Target Heart Rate") is recommended for all but the highly trained athlete. (Since body temperature can also rise in hot tubs, saunas, and whirlpools, avoid them or limit your bathing time to no more than 5 minutes.)

You can resume exercising after a normal vaginal delivery as soon as you have been given consent by your doctor. It is generally easier to recover from childbirth if you establish a regular exercise regime. Exercise can help restore those abdominal muscles that don't just pop back into shape without effort (Figure 2.7). Choose any physical activity as long as it doesn't cause pain. The only exception is swimming, which can cause bacterial infection, because the cervix needs time to close.

EXERCISE AND AGING

For a woman entering or past the age of menopause, exercising may be the single best thing she can do for her emotional and physical health. Whether or not she takes estrogen replacement, the active post-menopausal woman has a much better chance of keeping her heart healthy, her bones strong, and her body fit than her more sedentary sisters (Figure 2.8). The woman over 60 who exercises at least 30 minutes three times per week has the heart, lungs, and muscles of the woman ten years younger.

It can actually be dangerous to your health *not* to

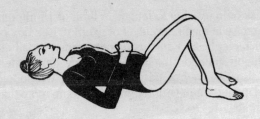

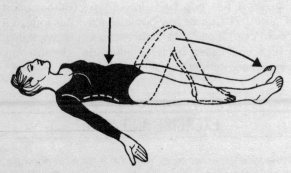

Figure 2.6. Abdominal Stretches. Stretching and strengthening the abdominal muscles is safe during the early part of pregnancy. All of these stretches are begun lying down with your hips, shoulders, and feet flat on the floor and your knees bent. **Top left: Back presses:** Press your lower back into the floor without raising your hips or shoulders; hold and release, then repeat. **Bottom left: Leg lifts:** Lift your feet off the floor and slowly straighten your legs all the way out and down. Then lift up your feet and bring your knees up again into the original position. To prevent lower back strain, be sure to use your abdomen, not your lower back, to raise and lower your legs during this exercise.

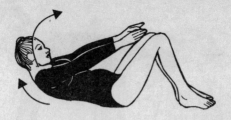

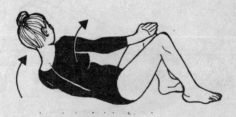

Top right: Straight curl-ups: Tuck in your chin and reach your hands up to your knees, allowing your shoulders to lift off the floor. Keep your lower back in contact with the floor during this exercise.
Bottom right: Reach with your right hand up and over to your left knee, keeping your left shoulder on the floor. Repeat on the other side.

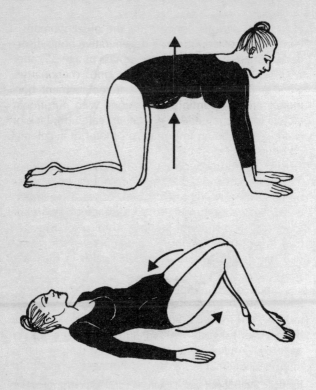

Figure 2.7. Abdominal muscles can be firmed up and returned to their normal shape after delivery by exercises that strengthen the muscles in the pelvis.
Top: Tummy tucks: On all fours with your hands directly beneath your shoulders and your knees under your hips, tIghten your abdominal muscles by rounding your back and curling inward.
Bottom: Pelvic tilts: Lie on your back with your knees bent and your feet on the floor. Press down on your lower back by contracting abdominal muscles; tilt your hips upward.

exercise. A serious concern for the older woman is the threat of osteoporosis, a degenerative bone disorder. Women reach a peak bone mass at age 35, after which bone gradually decreases until menopause, when a rapid decrease occurs if replacement hormones are not administered. Along with nutritional factors (not eating adequate dietary calcium), lack of exercise may be an important promoter of accelerated bone loss.

In addition, women well past the age of menopause may be able to increase their bone mass by performing weight-bearing exercises. Remember, even if you are returning to exercise after a period of inactivity, you are not starting from zero. Muscles may in fact have "memory." Being active in any way will do a lot to improve overall health in the later years.

Since older joints become stiff and inflexible there may be a need to do a longer warm-up and modify your exercise—perhaps by doing fewer repetitions. Work at your own target heart rate (see box on page 61). And always be alert to any danger signs: lightheadedness, chest pain, or shortness of breath. In terms of specific exercises, calisthenics promote flexibility, weightlifting promotes muscle strength, brisk walking is beneficial and convenient; and stationary bicycling and swimming strengthen the heart muscles and bones. Jogging may not be a good choice: the jogger's foot lands with a force equal to several times body weight, which can injure older bones, tendons, ligaments, and joints.

Again, it's never too late to start exercising. A 1987 survey on exercise, diet, and bone loss in the

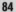

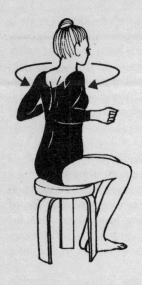

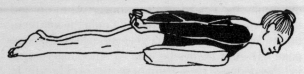

Figure 2.8. Back-Strengthening Exercises. Strengthening your back muscles can help avoid the back pain that often accompanies aging.
Top: To strengthen the trapezius muscles in the upper back and shoulders, sit with your back straight and your feet on the floor. With your arms relaxed and bent, pull back your shoulders as far as they will go.
Bottom: Lie face down with a cushion under your hips and torso, your arms at your sides, and your legs straight. Lift your head and feet off the floor at the same time and hold, then relax and repeat.

Journal of the American Geriatrics Society found that sedentary nursing home residents in their eighties experienced more than a 4 percent increase in density of the forearm bone when they performed mild exercises three times a week for three years. A group of nonexercisers underwent a 2.5 percent decline in bone density over the same time period.

Exercise will also help you maintain your weight or lose weight, even as your metabolism slows as you age. Not only will staying fit directly help you avoid developing serious diseases, such as diabetes and heart disease, but by exercising you will look and feel younger and more energetic. You may find that exercising alleviates some menopausal symptoms such as annoying hot flashes, and that your complexion looks and feels younger as more blood is pumped into the tiny capillaries that feed the skin. Improved circulation will also help your digestive system stay healthy and keep your immune system strong.

It's no wonder that the National Institutes of Health refer to exercise as "the most effective anti-aging pill ever discovered."

No one has found the fountain of youth—but you can certainly increase your odds and live longer and better by exercising. Staying physically fit should be a lifetime commitment.

PART 3
Living in a Healthy Environment

Diane L. Adams, M.D., M.P.H.

Our home environment has numerous health risks, many with the potential to cause health problems. There are potential biological hazards inside, such as mold or fungi, and outside, such as ticks that carry Lyme disease; there are physical hazards in and around the home, such as broken steps that could eventually collapse, or even a violent thunderstorm, with damaging winds and hail. Many of these hazards are easy to do something about; others are difficult for the individual to counteract. Being aware of the ones that can be dealt with is the first step toward improving health in and around the home.

Not all health hazards around the home lead to a health problem. In fact, most physical, biological, or chemical hazards can easily be coped with through proper use, cleanliness, and, in the case of chemicals, careful use and following of manufacturer's instructions. Ultimately, the majority of health problems caused by the effects of our surrounding environment—from inside the home to the backyard—can be controlled by our own choices.

BIOLOGICAL RISKS AROUND THE HOME

Microorganisms, such as viruses and bacteria, can be biological risks in and around the home. Most are harmless, while others can cause allergies, colds, and other respiratory ailments. Tiny organisms that cause respiratory ailments can be spread from person to person by air, water, bodily fluids; in most cases, allergens are carried by dust through the air. Molds and fungi can form from excess humidity and cause upper respiratory problems as they lodge in the lungs. Even setting out meats and certain foods on the counter for long periods of time invites microorganisms: *Campylobacter jejuni* (a bacteria that infects poultry, beef, and lamb) and *Staphylococcus aureus* (a common bacterium) are two disease-causing bacteria that proliferate under such conditions and can cause food poisoning.

There are other biological concerns outdoors, including plants and bugs. The best way to cope with the potential health risks from them is to be aware of the hazards.

Outdoor Biological Hazards

- *Poisonous Common Wild Plants:* Many plants are poisonous—do not eat any plant unless you are sure it is not poisonous. In particular, keep chldren from eating such plants as nightshade, wild mushrooms (to be safe, never eat any wild mushrooms), oak tree leaves and acorns, pokeweed, May apples (especially the fruit), and horse chestnuts. (See Fig. 3.1 A-D)

- *Poison Ivy, Poison Oak, Poison Sumac:* Up to 80% of the population is allergic to the oils in the leaves, roots, and stems of these plants. The oils cause itchy rashes and blisters if they are touched (the oils can also be on clothes if you brush past the leaves). For outbreaks of poison ivy, oak, or sumac (sumacs are only found in

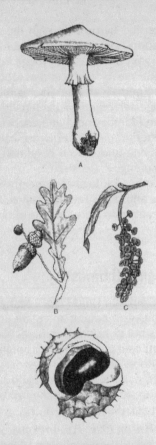

Figure 3.1. Some common wild plants are poisonous if eaten. Wild mushrooms (A) should never be eaten under any circumstances, even if you believe you know what species they are. Accidental poisonings and deaths can occur in experts who are knowledgeable about mushroom species. Oak tree leaves and acorns (B), pokeweed (C), especially the berries, and horse chestnuts (D) are also poisonous if eaten.

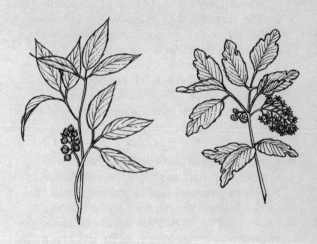

Figure 3.2.   Poison ivy (left) and poison oak (right) are abundant species that exude an oil (urushiol) from the stems and leaves that causes painful rashes upon contact. The oil can be carried on clothes, shoes, or pets that touch these plants.

the eastern United States), consult your doctor, who will probably prescribe a special lotion and medication if necessary. (See Fig. 3.2). In addition, do not scratch the rash or blisters. You risk infecting the damaged skin.

■ *Poisonous Common Garden Plants:* While most garden plants are harmless, there are some (plants, fruits, or leaves) that are poisonous to eat (unless noted, all the plant and its parts are poisonous): geranium, English Ivy, hyacinths (bulbs), daffodils, Lily-of-the-Valley, yew (seeds within the berry), rhododendron (even the honey from the flowers can make you ill), morning glory (seeds), holly (berries), mistletoe, tomatoes (vine and leaves), potatoes (green spots and sprouts—even cooking does not destroy the poison in the green spots), and seeds (also called pits) of most fruits (cherries, apples, peaches, plums, and apricots). (See Fig. 3.3).

■ *Common Insects and Outdoor Creatures to Watch:* Most backyards have no real harmful insects or creatures (unless you are allergic to certain bites or stings); most of the insects just cause irritating bites. With thousands of species of insects and outdoor creatures, it is impossible to list all those that can be obnoxious or dangerous. A very general list follows, and many of the insects and creatures overlap from one part of the country to the other (you can find out about other types of harmful insects in your area by contacting the cooperative extension service (USDA) in your locality):

Around the Country

■ *mosquitoes:* A mosquito bite causes an irritating, itchy welt (use over-the-counter anti-sting medication to stop the itching); in the tropics, mosquitos can carry malaria and yellow fever. (See Fig. 3.4).

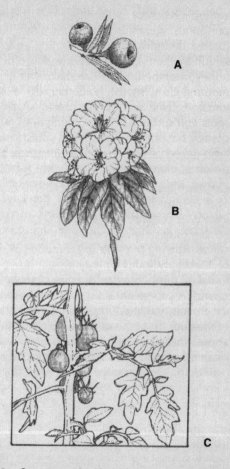

Figure 3.3.   Common garden plants that are poisonous if eaten include the berries of the yew (A), any part of a rhododendron (B), even the honey from the flowers, and the vine and leaves of the tomato (C).

- *bee, wasp, and hornet stings:* Bee, wasp, and hornet stings can cause a large irritating, itchy welt. The stinger may also be left in the skin (remove with tweezers). Those who are allergic to bee stings should see a doctor immediately after being stung (some people allergic to such stings carry medication with them when they are outdoors). To stop the itching, use over-the-counter anti-sting medication. (See Fig. 3.5).

- *flies (greenbottle, bluebottle, and houseflies are most common):* These flies do not sting (black-horse, deer, and black flies do—see below), but can spread filth and disease if they land on exposed food. They lay their eggs anywhere—on manure, garbage, or carcasses. Try to keep flies away from food at picnics or inside the house. (See Fig. 3.6).

- *snakes:* Although most species of snakes are harmless, there are several in various parts of the country that are poisonous. For instance, in the south, water moccasins (cottonmouths) and coral snakes are poisonous. To avoid snakes, be careful around open spaces in rock or wood piles and along garden paths. See a doctor immediately if you are bitten by a snake. (See Fig. 3.7).

Northeast

- *deer, black, and blackhorse flies:* The bites cause large, irritating, itchy welts; some people will have allergic reactions to such bites (consult a doctor if excessive swelling occurs).

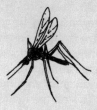

Figure 3.4.   The bite of the common mosquito can cause an irritating, itchy welt; in tropical areas, mosquitoes may carry malaria.

Figure 3.5.   Bee stings are painful and, in people who are severely allergic, can be dangerous or fatal. Shown here is a honeybee, one of the least aggressive bee species that can deliver a painful sting if disturbed.

- *deer ticks:* Deer ticks suck blood from their hosts. They are found in the woods (usually in deer territory, thus the name) from the spring to fall, peaking in the summer months. Some deer ticks carry Lyme disease, a bacterial infection that often begins as a simple rash (another symptom may or may not be a bullseye rash, flu-like symptoms, and muscle pain). If you find

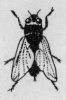

Figure 3.6. Houseflies are extremely common. Although they don't sting or bite, they can spread disease.

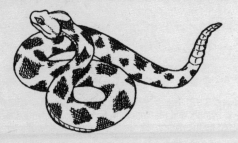

Figure 3.7. Most snakes found in the wild are harmless, but among those that aren't are some species of rattlesnakes. Depending on the species, a rattlesnake bite can cause a range of serious reactions, from respiratory distress to death.

a tick (they are usually about ¹/₈ inch or smaller in diameter), use tweezers and pull the tick straight out (do not twist). Put the tick in a bottle, and contact your doctor. (See Fig. 3.8).

Southeast

■ *ticks:* Many ticks in the Southeast (and some to the west) carry Rocky Mountain spotted fever. If

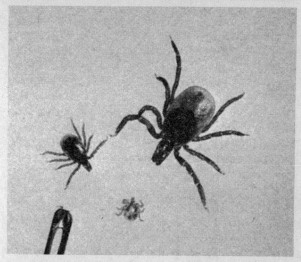

Figure 3.8.   The deer tick has three stages of development: larva, nymph, and mature adult. Most cases of lyme disease are caused by the nymph. Because it is only the size of a pin head, the nymph is difficult to see or feel, and it is most active in the spring and summer, when people are outside.

you find a tick (they are usually brown with spots on the back, and about ¹⁄₄ inch in diameter—an engorged tick may be up to ¹⁄₂ inch in diameter), use tweezers and pull the tick straight out (do not twist). Put the tick in a bottle, and contact your doctor. (See Fig. 3.9).

■ *fire ants:* Fire ants give painful stings, causing an irritating, itchy welt (use over-the-counter anti-sting medication to stop the itching). In particular, watch children playing in the backyard—they can be badly stung by a nest of fire ants.

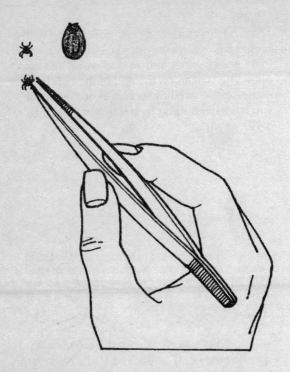

Figure 3.9. Ticks swell to many times their normal size (top right) when engorged with a host's blood. They should be removed by grasping them with tweezers (bottom) and pulling straight out, without twisting.

Southwest

- *scorpion:* Scorpions, about an inch long with a curled tail, have a very painful sting. Watch for them under stones and around wood and rock piles. The stinger, on the end of the tail, can cause severe swelling; contact your doctor if you have been stung by a scorpion. (See Fig. 3.10).

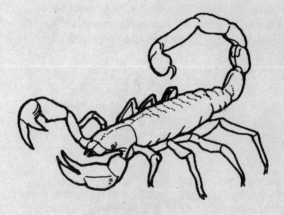

Figure 3.10.   Nine species of scorpion inhabit the United States. Most are found in the Southwest, but they range as far north as Idaho and as far east as Colorado. Few are dangerously poisonous, but the sting of at least one species can be fatal.

Indoor Biological Hazards

- *Common Poisonous Plants:* Although most indoor plants are harmless, there are several plants that are poisonous to eat, including poinsettia, philodendron leaves, dieffenbachia (or dumbcane) leaves, and Jerusalem cherry. (See Fig. 3.11).

- *Common Insects to Watch:* Common indoor insects can come from outdoors, or from insects that are found on humans and animals.

- *bed bugs:* Bed bugs are found in rugs or bedding. At night, they crawl (they never fly or jump) to feed on humans or animals. They are smaller than ¹/₄ inch in diameter and are

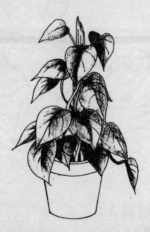

Figure 3.11. The philodendron, a common houseplant, is poisonous if eaten by people or pets.

brownish, broad, and flat. Both males and females bite, leaving a painful rash of small welts. Bed bugs can be eliminated by washing linens; for more extensive cases, exterminators must be called in to eliminate the bugs.

- *fleas:* Fleas are most often carried by indoor animals. There are 1,000 different kinds of fleas, depending on the hosts (dogs, cats, mice, etc.). They have no wings, but can hop from about 8 to 13 inches. A flea bite can leave a painful rash of small welts. Fleas can be eliminated by using special flea sprays or by bug exterminators (to lower the risk of further infestation, have dogs, cats, and other animals wear flea collars). (See Fig. 3.12).

- *lice:* There are three types of lice found on humans: head, body, and crab. The lice are wingless, have brown to gray bodies, and cause an irritating itch. Head lice are found mostly in the scalp, or around any bodyhair; washing with special shampoo helps to eliminate head lice.

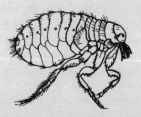

Figure 3.12.   Fleas can be carried indoors by dogs or cats, and their bites can cause welts or a rash on human skin.

Body lice occur in any part of the body; a special soap helps to eliminate most body lice.
Crab lice occupy certain hairy parts of the body, especially the groin area; they thrive in moist conditions. To eliminate crab lice, use a special soap.

- *dust mites:* Dust mites are microscopic creatures that live in the dust of your home. They live off particles in the home, most commonly human dead skin cells. They pose no real health threat unless you are allergic to the mites—allergic reactions include sneezing, runny nose, and cough.
  The best way to eliminate dust mites is to keep dust (including the notorious "dust bunnies") to a minimum by vacuuming and dusting.

PHYSICAL RISKS AROUND THE HOME

Many major risks around the home are physical, and are usually easily taken care of or repaired: broken stairs, loose electrical lines, or unsecured rugs. These hazards can lead to abrasions, fractures, lacerations, and burns. Protecting yourself from physical hazards in the home is mostly common sense: fix damaged stairs and broken floorboards to prevent tripping; use rugs with rubber backing to prevent slipping on smooth floors; hide loose wires and long cords to prevent tripping; and place rubber mats in the bathtub and rubber-backed rugs on the bathroom floor to stop slipping.

TERMS IN ENVIRONMENTAL HEALTH

In order to understand the potential dangers around us, it is necessary to understand the terms that are used in describing environmental conditions and health:

Allergens: Substances that cause physical reactions in persons sensitive to them through touch, inhalation, or ingestion. The most common forms of allergens are from dust, pollen, animal dander, and insect parts.

Carcinogens: Carcinogens are cancer-causing chemical compounds. Exposure to a carcinogen does not mean that a person will develop cancer, but that the risk for cancer increases. For example, tobacco has a mixture of carcinogens, and people who smoke have a higher risk of developing a number of different cancers.

Contaminants: In reference to pollution, contaminants are chemical substances that change the composition of the air, water, and soils by their presence and may or may not affect humans in an adverse way. It is often used interchangeably with *pollutant;* although a pollutant is usually a harmful substance, whereas a contaminant may not be harmful.

Epidemiological studies: Epidemiological studies look at groups of people in the same (or similar) localities to determine existing reasons for a health problem within the group.

For example, looking at clusters of cancers within a community may help determine why certain cancers are prevalent and identify the cause.

Exposure: Exposure is defined as coming into contact with a health hazard, which may or may not affect the human body. Exposures to potential health risks can be one-time occurrences or a number of occurrences over an extended duration. The human body's reaction can be immediate, or a period of time may elapse between the exposure and onset of the health problem. A continual high- or low-level exposure to a hazard can also lead to a health problem after a long period of time, such as long exposure to excessive amounts of natural radon gas, which has been linked to lung cancer in some people.

Hazard: An event, structure, or substance that has potential to harm the human body in some way. Major hazards can be physical, biological, or chemical. For example, chemical hazards include carcinogens (chemicals that cause cancers), teratogens (chemicals that cause birth defects), and toxins (chemicals that are harmful or fatal to humans in low doses).

Pesticides: Pesticides are chemicals used to eliminate pests from commercial or residental crops or from homes. There are thousands of pesticides known to exist, many of which are not banned or registered with the Environmental Protection Agency. Pesticides are divided into several groups: insecticides (which kill insects), herbicides (which kill plants), fungicides (which kill fungi), and rodenticides (which kill rodents).

Particulate matter: Very small pieces or particles of substances in the air we breathe, including smoke, soot, ash, dust (includes human dander and microscopic insect parts), and aerosol sprays. Particulate matter comes from many sources, including industrial processes, burning of fuels, volcanoes, dust storms, aerosol cans, burning of vegetation and wood; it occurs as residue from grinding, quarrying, demolition, and milling operations; and it is associated with some homebased hobbies, such as woodworking.

Radiation: Radiation is the emission of energy in the form of certain electromagnetic rays, including microwaves, ultraviolet light, and X-rays. The sun is the greatest source of naturally occurring radiation, but radiation is also produced by man-made sources such as microwave ovens and power lines.

Risk: A risk is the perceived harm an event, substance, or entity can have on a human. Risk usually has to do with statistics and the population; that is, what percentage of the population would be affected by the exposure to a potential hazard and the resulting health problems from such an exposure. It is difficult to interpret risk based on a hazard's effects on people because everyone responds differently to an exposure. Although there are some hazards known to affect all humans in relatively the same way, everyone is chemically different: Some people may be more genetically inclined toward being affected by a substance, and some can tolerate a greater exposure than others.

Toxin: Toxins are any substances that are harmful or fatal to humans at a high enough dosage. There are thousands of potential toxins, for many of which it has been difficult to evaluate the health hazards. The level of a toxic dose of each toxic substance is difficult to pinpoint, as the toxic dose to a human is usually derived from animal studies or from the health records of individuals actually exposed to the substances.

Other physical risks are found outside the home, including improper use of lawn machines (lawnmowers, electric hedge clippers), and tripping on uneven walkways or stairs. Sunburn—caused by the burning of the skin by the ultraviolet rays of the sun—is a major risk because of its link to skin cancer, especially in fair-skinned people. The average number of skin cancer deaths each year is 8,500 (and many researchers believe it is on the rise because of the destruction of atmospheric ozone). People can reduce their chances of skin cancer by wearing light protective clothing and sunscreens, preferably with a sun-protection factor (SPF) of 15 or higher.

CHEMICAL RISKS AROUND THE HOME

Chemicals in the environment are all around us and are virtually inescapable. Chemicals are found in and on the foods we buy at the store; in our clothing, cosmetics, and furniture; and in the air, water, and soil. Most of these chemicals create few problems for human health. Others cause health problems ranging from allergies and skin rashes to cancer and poisoning.

Chemicals can affect health immediately over the short-term or cumulatively as chemicals build up in the body. Some chemicals appear to have a particular effect on women, especially those who are pregnant or in their childbearing years; other chemicals affect women, men, and children alike. The following list describes the chemicals that are of most concern to us in and around our homes, and possible symptoms of exposure (an asterisk [*] marks those chemicals that are common in many homes):

Arsenic: Arsenic is a highly poisonous metallic element when digested, although long ago people ate small quantities daily for medicinal reasons with no ill effect. Arsenic is found in weed killers, insecticides, and in combinations of metals. It is of most concern to families living around mines and in rural areas where use of insecticides is widespread. Symptoms of arsenic exposure include nausea, vomiting, restlessness, darkening of the skin, headaches, memory loss, and convulsions. Arsenic has also been linked to cancer of the lungs and liver. *If you suspect that you have been exposed to arsenic, see your doctor immediately.*

Asbestos Fibers: Asbestos is a fire retardant and was once (and still is, in some cases) used in brake linings, hair dryers, fireproof fabrics, asphalt, shingles, pipe insulation, and home insulation. In 1980, after asbestos was reported to cause lung cancer in asbestos workers and mesotheliomas in people living near asbestos plants, the Environmental Protection Agency promoted the removal of asbestos from buildings. Recent studies have shown that such removal may not have been necessary: more problems occurred when the asbestos material broke up on removal. In addition, the wastes from the removal process were difficult to get rid of, as landfills were closing or refusing to allow asbestos on site.

*Carbon Monoxide: Carbon monoxide is the odorless, colorless gas that is released in car exhaust; from a kerosene heater or stove; in vapors released when stripping paint or varnish with methylene chloride; or in cigarette, pipe, and cigar smoke. It is also one of the leading causes of death by poisoning in the United States. Carbon monoxide can enter the bloodstream by inhaling or skin absorption, the gas attaching itself to the hemoglobin in red blood cells and preventing oxygen from reaching vital parts of the body. Symptoms of low dosage include headache, lethargy, nausea, and fainting; higher amounts can lead to bizarre behavior, and for prolonged periods, it may be fatal, as the body is "starved" of oxygen. If you suspect carbon monoxide poisoning, get to fresh air as soon as possible (open a window, or go outdoors). Keep kerosene heaters or stoves in proper working condition; use paint strippers or varnishes in a well-ventilated area; and use air filters to filter out

cigarette, pipe, and cigar smoke (or stop smoking).

Carbon Tetrachloride: Carbon tetrachloride is a solvent and cleaner found in many households and has been widely used for many years. It is a known liver toxin as well as a hepatocarcinogen (cause of liver cancer); it is also considered a central nervous system depressant.

*Dust and Particulate Matter: Dust is all around us, and it carries particulate matter in the form of molds, bacteria, mites, soil, gases, lead, soot, and ash. Small amounts of particulate matter are common in most households, usually entering the house through open windows or air conditioning units. Larger amounts of particles are more of a concern for those living near quarries, mines, dusty fields, or demolition sites. Some hobbies are also associated with larger particles, including home machine shops and woodworking. Smaller particulate matter inside or outside of the home is of particular concern to those who have allergies to mites, molds, or pollen. Dust may also hold lead particles, often from lead paint from older buildings, which in excess can lead to health problems. Long-term exposure to certain types of dust may cause scarring (fibrosis) of the lungs, resulting in shortness of breath (called pneumoconiosis), although this condition is usually found in association with those who work in certain fields, such as sandblasting, mining, or welding. If you are concerned that you have a health problem associated with dust or particulate materials, try purchasing an air filter for your home; air conditioners often eliminate dust from the outside but should be properly maintained. For hobbies that create larger particles,

wear protective face masks and have proper ventilation. If your condition worsens (especially upper respiratory problems), see your doctor.

Fluorocarbons: Fluorocarbons are chemical compounds of carbon and fluorine. They are most often found in solvents and as propellants in spray cans, lubricants, and insulators. Inhalation of fluorocarbons, especially in spray cans, can cause nausea or even unconsciousness. To eliminate possible contamination by fluorocarbons, use all chemicals in a well-ventilated area, and follow manufacturers' suggestions for use.

Food Chemicals: Many of our foods contain certain chemicals that can be harmful, especially in excess. Cured meat, smoked fish, and some beers contain sodium nitrite to prevent bacterial growth associated with botulism; but when sodium nitrite combines with nitrosamine, found in other foods, it becomes carcinogenic. Other chemicals are in foods as additives, preservatives, and flavorings. Most that have been proven to be harmful to humans have been banned from use; others have a negative health effect on people who are sensitive to the chemicals. In most cases, it is up to the consumer to decide what chemicals they want to avoid. If you realize you have an adverse reaction to a chemical, read labels and avoid products that would cause you to react.

Formaldehyde: Formaldehyde is found in fabrics (clothing, drapes, rugs, and upholstery); both the home and car contain the chemical. It is also used in particle board, plywood, and some foam insulation (it was banned from use in insulation in 1982, but older homes may still have such insulation).

Formaldehyde is a suspected carcinogen; in excess, it is an irritant to smell and can hurt the nasal membranes, eyes, throat, and lungs. To lower the risk of exposure to formaldehyde (especially fumes), wash new fabrics; choose other types of paneling, not particle board or plywood (when purchasing such products, ask how the wood was processed); open the window after installing new rugs; and vacuum new cloth-covered furniture. If you still suspect that formaldehyde is a problem, seek medical attention.

Lead: Lead is a known poisonous element. It is used to line storage tanks and pipes; it is also used in batteries. Certain types of industry release lead in particulate form from smokestacks, although there are strict government laws that regulate the amounts released.

Exposure to lead in the home is usually from the air from nearby industry. Hobbyists who make ceramics (glazes), solder stained glass, or target shoot are all exposed to higher levels of lead. Although it was banned from paints in the last decade, there are still homes with old lead paint on the walls. Such paint poses the most serious threat to children and animals, who tend to eat the pieces of the paint that flake from the walls.

Lead can hurt a fetus, whose nervous system is vulnerable to the toxic effects of lead; exposure to the metal can cause permanent learning disabilities, hyperactivity, and mental disorders in children. The metal is particularly harmful to young children, who often exhibit learning disabilities after long-term exposure; in adults, lead exposure can cause irritability and mental confusion. Highest doses can cause severe brain damage and death. *If you suspect lead poisoning, see your doctor immediately (there are blood tests that can be administered to determine lead levels in the blood).*

Mercury: Mercury is a poisonous heavy metal similar to lead. It is used in chemical pesticides, barometers and thermometers, mercury lamps, antiseptics, and germicides. Photographers are exposed to mercury in the development process; painters who use certain pigments in paints also are exposed to small amounts of mercury; metalworkers are susceptible to mercury poisoning, either by direct contact or by breathing particles of mercury. Seafood lovers should also be concerned about mercury: in 1976, dumping of mercury into waterways was banned because fish had particularly high levels of the chemical in their bodies. The concern was not the fish (they are not affected by the metal), but to humans who ate the fish.

Mercury poisoning has many symptoms. Organic mercurials cause dizziness, slurred speech, diarrhea, and convulsions; inhaling mercury oxide fumes cause flu-like symptoms. Mercury is readily absorbed into the skin when touched; never try to pick up the mercury from a broken thermometer with your bare hands. A major debate is whether mercury amalgam used in dental fillings is a health problem. The choice of using mercury amalgam for fillings is the consumer's choice; if you suspect exposure to mercury, seek medical attention.

Perchloroethylene: Perchloroethylene is the chemical you smell when you enter a dry cleaning establishment. It is a central nervous system depressant and can cause dizziness and nausea in some people. It has also been found to cause cancer in animals, but such a connection to humans has not been proven.

Polychlorinated Biphenyls (PCBs): Almost all living things have PCBs in their tissues. These chemical compounds have been used in generators, transformers, and large electrical equipment for years; in 1979, because they were suspected of being carcinogenic, PCBs were banned from use in equipment. Even so, other countries still use PCBs in the manufacture of lubricants, adhesives, and solvents. The problem with PCBs is their long lives: they take years to break down into a harmless substance. PCBs are soluble in the fatty tissue of humans and animals and remain for years in the body, but little is known about their effects on the body. It is unlikely that PCBs will be a problem within the home, but there are still some areas that have not eliminated transformers or other electrical equipment with PCBs. In most states, PCB-containing equipment must have warning signs that the substance is in use.

Polyvinyl Chloride (PVC): PVC is found in the plastics that surround us: credit cards, furniture, shower curtains, computers, cars, garden hoses, and some plumbing pipes. It is a known carcinogen, and the particles can be harmful if you file, cut, or sandpaper plastics containing PVC; such work should be conducted in a well-ventilated area, and a face mask should be worn.

Radon: Radon is a colorless, odorless gas that occurs naturally from the decay of radioactive elements (especially uranium). It is found everywhere in the soil, including material made from soils, such as brick, stone, adobe, tile, concrete, and cinder blocks. The distribution of the gas varies throughout the country, being more abundant where uranium exists underground. In very large amounts, radon can cause lung cancer over time. Smaller amounts appear to do no appreciable harm.

Tobacco Smoke: More than 4,000 chemical compounds—mostly irritants and carcinogens (about 43 of them are carcinogens)—have been identified in cigarette smoke, including carbon monoxide, benzene, nitrosamines, nicotine, and nitrogen dioxide. Smoking has been linked to lung cancer and emphysema in smokers and a range of ailments in those exposed to secondhand smoke, especially children. Children of smokers suffer from a higher incidence of respiratory infections than children of nonsmoking parents; 6- to 11-year-olds who live around a parent who smoked had lower heights and weights than children from households with nonsmoking parents. If you are concerned that you have any health problem associated with cigarettes, stop smoking. If your condition worsens, see your doctor.

Trichloroethane and Trichloroethylene: Trichloroethane is used as a chemical intermediary for hundreds of products and in aerosol waterproofing sprays. Trichloroethylene was widely used as a degreaser. Both chemicals are known to be central nervous system depressants.

HOW TO HELP YOUR HOME ENVIRONMENT

Healthy Air

Although most air in and around the home falls within safety standards, it can contain carbon monoxide, particulates, sulfur oxides, nitrous oxides, and photochemical oxidants from nearby industry or cities. Inside, pollutants can come from cigarette smoke, furniture, carpeting, certain interior structural materials (such as pressboard), household chemical products, and radon. Outside, air pollutants come from auto exhaust, emissions from fossil fuel power plants, industrial processes, and forest fires.

Smog is probably the major outdoor air pollutant. Smog is the result of a chemical reaction caused by sunlight acting on hydrocarbons (methane, benzene, and other products of combustion), nitrogen oxides, and other pollutants. The results include ground-level ozone, aldehydes, ketones, peroxyacetyl nitrates, organic acids, and sulfuric acids (a source of acid rain). Carbon oxides, sulfur oxides, and particulate matter are also prevalent as air pollutants.

Inside the Home

1. Tobacco: Tobacco is one of the largest single sources of indoor air pollution. Recent studies have shown that passive smoking, or breathing someone else's smoke from cigarettes, cigars, and pipes, can also increase a bystander's chance of contracting lung cancer or developing respiratory ailments. Quitting smoking immediately can avoid future health problems and allow your body to recover from previous intake of tobacco and the bystanders smoke.

2. Furnishings: The best way to lower the problem with formaldehyde is to have adequate ventilation and wash fabrics to eliminate much of the formaldehyde fumes.

3. Radon: There are simple radon kits on the market that will measure the amount of radon in your home. In many states, the health department can tell you more about your choices. The interest in energy conservation in the 1970s, which included making homes airtight and energy efficient, may have exacerbated the levels of radon in homes. Since it is impossible to prevent radon from occurring, the best way to cope with elevated levels is to improve circulation within the home, repair cracks in the basement floor or walls, and vent the gas to the outside.

4. Household Products: Substitute water-based or "environmentally safe" household products for the home; others may contain hydrocarbon gases that could cause upper respiratory ailments. Do not combine cleaning products (or any other household products) unless suggested by the manufacturer. Especially dangerous is the combination of bleach and ammonia. These chemicals react with each other and can cause upper respiratory ailments, fainting, or even damage to the lungs.

5. Filtering the Air: Air filters may be the answer to cleaning the air sufficiently to eliminate possible particulates from your home. Air cleaners often help people who have asthma attacks and allergies from pollen or dust. Air conditioners may also help people with allergies; but caution must be taken to keep the air conditioner clean to prevent disease-causing bacteria and mold.

Outside the Home

1. Smog: Smog is the biggest concern outside the home. Smog alerts—when air quality degrades to dangerous levels—often occur when hot, humid high pressure systems stagnate over a region. The weather system acts like a cap, holding the smog over the area; the smog increases as cars, industry, and other processes continue to pump chemicals into the air. During smog alerts reduce your activity (to decrease the amount of smog entering the lungs); remain indoors when possible and keep windows closed or partially closed; keep an eye on children, the elderly, and people with respiratory ailments, and advise them to stay inside.

2. Electromagnetic Fields: Electromagnetic fields (EMFs) are of major concern to those who live near high-power electrical wires. The effects of the EMFs are questionable, but in 1990 the Environmental Protection Agency announced that EMFs were "possible" human carcinogens because of several reports that linked electromagnetic fields with leukemia, lymphoma, and brain cancer in children; adult health problems were only in association with working in the electrical fields. The information on EMFs is contradictory: one recent study suggested that women who work in the electrical trades run a 38 percent greater risk of dying from breast cancer than other working women, yet other studies show no such connection between human health risk and EMFs.

TOO MUCH NOISE

One of the most ignored, yet troublesome, environmental health problems is noise pollution. It does not involve particulates or dangerous chemicals; noise pollution is caused by sound that can cause damage to the ears, increase stress, and may lead to behavioral problems.

Excessive noise—mainly associated with large cities (vehicles are the major source), airports, and recreational noise—can cause damage to the ears: tinnitus (ringing in the ears, which can occur for years even after exposure to one loud noise); loss of high-, middle-, or low-pitch hearing; and physical damage to the eardrum. Case study upon case study has shown that noise does cause certain levels of stress, anxiety, and insomnia in some individuals, depending on the person and loudness and pitch of the noise. Loud noise can lead to physiological changes, such as hypertension (high blood pressure); some sounds can be addictive (sounds from "boom boxes" could elevate levels of adrenaline in the body); and certain behavior has been reported to be caused by noise.

The simplest way to reduce your exposure to noise in the home is to turn down the volume to radios, televisions, and stereos. Bothersome noise coming from outside the home can often be subdued by "white noise," a soft, constant noise to block out the outdoor sounds, for example, radio static. Protect your ears from loud noises, especially in hobbies such as boating, snowmobiling, and hunting. Protective earmuffs or earplugs can protect you from ear damage.

Healthy Water

About 90 percent of the U.S. population relies on city water supplies, which are monitored for safety and contaminants. City water is usually not subject to contamination. There are many sources of water pollution, including leaking gasoline tanks and landfills, pesticides, chemical dumping (often illegally in rivers, lakes, and oceans and along highways), and vehicle and industrial emissions. Every source of water on the planet—groundwater, lakes, oceans, rivers, and streams—contains some type of pollution, which may or may not cause health problems. The threat of water pollution is mainly to rural private wells, which get their water from groundwater sources; and many of the sources are close to agricultural centers, landfills, or dumps.

Inside the Home

1. Test Water: It is important to be aware of possible contamination; people with wells near landfills, agricultural fields, and old chemical plants or dumps should be particularly watchful. Contact the local health department for possible contamination reports around your home. If you have any suspicion of contamination, hire independent state-certified laboratories for testing (not laboratories that sell water treatment equipment, as their results may not be objective). Test the water at least once a year in any case. Test for contaminants such as organic and inorganic chemicals, radon, and bacteria. To interpret the test results, consult the office of the Environmental Protection Agency near you.

2. Keep Water: If your city or town reports water contamination, be sure to follow the health department's directions (including boiling water); if harsher contaminants are found, do not drink the water or use it for bathing, as per the direction of the health department. Those who live near flood-prone areas should keep extra jugs of water in storage in case of emergency; change the water frequently to keep it fresh.

3. Lead from Pipes: There are several ways to lower the presence of lead in the water: do not use hot tap water for cooking or drinking (hot water dissolves lead in the plumbing more readily); let water run from the tap for about 30 seconds before taking a drink, for about 3 minutes in the morning, and for about 5 to 7 minutes after more than a week-long vacation, as lead levels are higher in standing water in pipes.

Outside the Home

1. Dumping Pollutants: One of the ways to prevent contamination of water supplies (especially in rural areas where most homes use wells for drinking, bathing, and cooking water) is not to dump pollutants in gutters, in the backyard, or in rivers, lakes, or streams. Contaminants such as motor oil or concentrated lawn chemicals should be disposed of at specified recycling centers.

2. Pesticides and Lawn Care: Another way in which groundwater is contaminated is by the excessive use of pesticides and lawn care chemicals, especially in rural areas that depend on groundwater for their water supplies. A solution is to use organic alternatives to pesticides; older pesticides and chemicals should be brought to specified recycling centers.

3. Septic Systems: Septic systems in rural areas should be installed by certified septic system companies. The systems should be located so as not to contaminate nearby water wells and must be sealed from corrosion, watched for leakage, and not allowed to overflow.

Healthy Land and Outdoors

Soils are of concern to many homeowners, as grounds can carry and hold toxins or chemicals for long periods of time. If soils are contaminated, there is a chance that young children playing in the yard, or even the avid gardener tending her flowers and vegetables, could be exposed to toxins.

Contamination of the soil may have many sources: chemicals from landfills leach into the soils; chemicals sprayed on gardens and lawns seep into the soil; old or used oil or chemicals are often wrongly thrown into the backyard or gutters; and emissions from industry, automobiles, and chemical plants deposit chemicals, heavy metals, and particulates into the soil.

Inside the Home

1. Recycling and Precycling: One way to cut back on what is sent to the landfills is to reuse or recycle newspapers, plastics, glass, cans, and other recyclable materials. Most of these materials do not decompose in the landfill for years, if at all, and may produce harmful chemicals that can leak into the soil and groundwater. Precycling is choosing products that use the least amount of disposable packaging.

2. Used Oils and Chemicals: Dispose of used oil at a recycling center or gas station—never dump it into the sewer system or in the backyard. Get rid of old, unusable chemicals (such as household cleaners, solvents, or pesticides) at special recycling centers or at chemical recycling drives held by local governments or environmental groups.

Outside the Home

1. Lead in Soils: A major concern is soil contaminated with lead. Chips or particles of old lead-based house paint is the most common source of the metal contaminant. Soils near busy roads may also contain lead from the days of leaded gas. Children playing in the soil near homes or around buildings can be exposed to toxic levels of lead. One of the best ways to avoid exposure to lead in the soil is not to let children play around flaking paint or close to the road of a busy street. Getting rid of lead in the soil is more difficult, requiring the expensive removal of the soils.

2. Testing the Soils: If you suspect your soil to be contaminated (for example, if you live near an old chemical plant or a major industry), have the grounds tested by a certified laboratory (look under "soil testing" in the telephone directory). The laboratory will also provide options if your soil is found to be contaminated.

3. Rural and Urban Pesticides and Chemical Sprays: Rural locations have an even more insidious problem with chemicals: agricultural fertilizer and pesticides that enter the soils. Urban lawns also commonly have pesticides. Because these chemicals can remain in the soil for a long time, modify their use and research more natural alternatives to the pesticides you use on your garden, bushes, trees, and lawn. Use alternatives to chemical fertilizers, especially natural composting.

Healthy Food

The most common concerns about the safety of food are residue pesticides, chemicals and additives, poor preparation, and raw foods.

Inside the Home

1. Clean Foods: To rid fruit and vegetables of pesticides and other contaminants, clean them with mild soap and water, then rinse. Purchase fruits and vegetables that were grown organically to lower your exposure to chemical pesticides.

2. What Is Added: Not all foods with additives or chemicals cause problems; the consumer must make her own decisions about the ingestion of additives and chemicals. In most cases, food additives have no adverse effects on people. The best way to protect yourself from possible health problems from additives and chemicals is to know how your body reacts to certain products.

3. Proper Handling: Be sure to refrigerate meats until they are ready to be prepared. The cold stops the growth of microbes, and proper cooking of food kills biological contaminants. Always clean your hands before handling any food. When handling meats, be sure to cut with a clean knife on a clean cutting board and cook with uncontaminated equipment. Common contaminants are the bacteria *Salmonella* and *Campylobacter,* both of which produce gastroenteritis, evidenced by vomiting and/or nausea. To control these bacteria, food should not be kept out of the refrigerator for more than 2 hours. Meats, eggs, and dairy products should be put in the refrigerator as soon as possible after use.

4. Raw Food: Eating raw food is not recommended, especially raw eggs, milk, fish, raw cheese, and meats. These foods are more susceptible to microbial contamination. For example, eggs may contain the *Salmonella* bacterium, which can cause food poisoning; cooking the eggs until they are solid (such as hard-boiling) kills the bacteria.

Outside the Home

1. Labels: When grocery shopping, read labels (now a law for most foods) to determine the additives, chemicals, and preservatives added to processed foods. Make your own decision as to the amounts of such chemicals you want you or your family to ingest.

SPECIAL CONCERNS FOR WOMEN

Beside avoiding hazards in the air, water, soil, and foods, women—especially those in their childbearing years—must watch for other hazardous exposures that could lead to health problems, mainly in the reproductive system. Of particular concern is the developing fetus, who is more susceptible to environmental hazards during the various stages of its life before birth.

Prenatal Conditions

There are several stages of fetal development when the fetus is most susceptible to agents that cause birth defects. During the first two weeks, certain hazards, mostly chemical, can cause the fertilized egg not to implant itself on the uterine wall. At this point, some chromosomal problems may occur from the exposure to the hazard, which may result in a spontaneous miscarriage.

At 3 to 8 weeks, the developing embryo forms most of the major organs. At this point, the fetus is very vulnerable to environmental teratogens (drugs that cause abnormal fetal development and are responsible for birth defects), which can interfere with, or even stop the functioning of, the formation of organ structures and could cause a miscarriage. In general, after the eighth week, environmental hazards have less of a physical effect on the fetus. But because the nervous system is still growing, certain environmental hazards can damage the fetus's mental development and lead to retardation. Of course, a major hazardous exposure, such as a massive dosage of radiation, would be harmful to both the mother and child.

The Fetus and Children at Risk

Most children are born healthy, even when born to mothers exposed to certain hazards in and around the home. As with adults, fetuses and children are affected by exposure to environmental hazards based on characteristics such as genetic susceptibility, the nature of the hazard, the dosage received, and the exposure time. It is estimated that 95 to 97 percent of children born in the United States each year have no sign of birth defects; of the 3 to 5 percent who do, about 2 to 10 percent of the birth defects are caused by chemical exposure, drugs, or environmental hazards.

There are certain "controllable" chemicals that a woman should be aware of during her pregnancy that have the potential to harm the fetus:

■ *Alcohol:* It is known that alcohol contains ethanol and acetaldehyde, two toxins that easily pass through the placenta to circulate in the fetus. Alcohol consumed during the first trimester, when fetal organs are forming, is the most damaging; and acetaldehyde is thought to contribute to the disruption of cell growth and metabolism. Researchers still do not know if moderate drinking (one to two drinks per day) has an negative effect on the fetus, but women are cautioned to avoid all alcohol consumption during pregnancy. Heavy or frequent drinkers face twice the risk of miscarriage; the child may have fetal alcohol syndrome, including delay in growth, abnormal features of the face and head, and nervous system abnormalities. A lesser effect from excessive alcoholic consumption during pregnancy is called fetal alcohol effect, which includes some eye and heart defects, impairment of certain organs, slowed growth, and behavioral problems such as hyperactivity and excessive irritability.

■ *Tobacco:* Women who smoke run the risk of adversely affecting not only their own health but also the growing fetus. Cigarettes increase the amount of carbon dioxide entering the fetal system, reducing oxygen to the growing baby. Some of the effects on the fetus appear to be smaller lung development (which may make the child more susceptible to respiratory ailments); smaller size; and premature birth. As to be expected, the more the cigarettes smoked per day, the greater the problems resulting in the fetus. There are also studies that connect passive, secondhand smoke to low birth weight, although these studies are not conclusive.

■ *Drugs:* Almost all recreational drugs (cocaine, marijuana, and heroin and other opiates) are connected with possible developmental effects in unborn children. Cocaine can remain in the fetus much longer than in an adult (sometimes a single dose lasting for five days); the affected baby is jittery, has low birth weight, and is usually born prematurely. Marijuana, like cigarettes, can reduce oxygen flow to the fetus; other studies, although not conclusive, show that affected babies have lower birth weights. The effects of heroin and other opiates are more difficult to determine—because in many of these cases other substances are also in use—but one of the major threats to babies born to heroin-using mothers is withdrawal: some 60 to 90 percent suffer from withdrawal, including tremors, fever, seizures, and irregular breathing. Most babies born to heroin addicts have serious medical problems, such as respiratory ailments and brain hemorrhages, and are at risk of having HIV (the virus that causes AIDS).

■ *Over-the-counter and Prescription Medications:* Medication can have an adverse effect on the growing fetus. Every pregnant woman should consult her doctor before taking any medication, even if it is an over-the-counter drug. In addition, if she believes she is pregnant, she should tell her doctor, dentist, or specialist— especially if her doctor is going to prescribe a medication. One of the best ways to determine if a drug may harm a fetus is to read the warnings on the medication bottle. If you are pregnant, it is best to consult your doctor before taking any medication, even for such medications as aspirin, cold and allergy medicines, and laxatives.

HEALTH WATCH

Federal, state, and local governments help in the regulation of hazards within our environment. If you are concerned about a possible health problem in or around your home and want to become involved in mitigating an environmental health problem, you may want to contact certain health services for information concerning the environmental health problem:

- *Public Health Service:* Public health departments inspect the meat, poultry, and fish industry for any violations of health regulations; keep restaurants, markets, and hospitals within health safety guidelines; and enforce regulations that are designed to prevent the contamination of food, drugs, beverages, and cosmetics. They include six major divisions: the National Institutes of Health (NIH), which provide funding for medical research studies; the Food and Drug Administration (FDA), which oversees the wholesomeness of the products (except meat, poultry, and eggs) consumed in the United States and are responsible for the control and prohibition of harmful chemicals (natural or synthetic) in food, drugs, and substances; the Centers for Disease Control and Prevention (CDC), a collection of centers that provide information on communicable diseases around the country and collect epidemiology studies of certain diseases; the Substance Abuse and Mental Health Services Administration (SAMHSA), which provides research and services aimed at reducing or controlling substance abuse and mental health problems; the Agency for Toxic Substances and Disease Registry (ATSDR), which prevents exposure to and adverse effects from hazardous substances; the Health Resources and Services Administration (HRSA), which oversees projects aimed at improving health services for mothers, infants, and children.

- *United States Department of Agriculture:* This federal government agency is responsible for the safety of meat, poultry, and eggs. It is responsible for the "USDA inspection" stickers often found on meats. The USDA Meat and Poultry hotline is 1-800-535-4555.

- *Environmental Protection Agency (EPA):* This federal government agency is in charge of protecting public health by controlling air and water. It is also in charge of regulating the production, use, and disposal of toxic chemicals in the environment.

- *State and Local Health Departments:* The state and local health departments have a variety of duties. Many state health departments disseminate information to the public concerning major environmental health concerns, such as radon gas. Cities or towns are in charge of sanitary engineering departments (including garbage collection and landfill maintenance) and sewage treatment (including sewage treatment plants and sewer lines).

PART 4
Working in a Healthy Environment

Rosemary K. Sokas, M.D., M.O.H., F.A.C.P.

What does work mean for a woman? Research has shown that women work longer hours for less money than men and devote a greater proportion of time, energy, and income to child rearing. At the same time, women in industrialized countries live longer than men; women working outside the home in these countries are also healthier and happier than those not in the paid work force. Work that is valued enables the individual to participate as a contributing member of society, achieve self-respect and financial security, and develop a network of supporting relationships.

The key word here is *value*, which is not synonymous with *money*; unpaid work in the home may be highly valued and provide all the personal benefits already mentioned. In our society, however, secure support systems and income security (including retirement benefits, health insurance, etc.) require conscious planning. Americans have traditionally assigned high worth to individualism and to material self-improvement, presenting additional hurdles for the woman who remains outside the paid work force. Finally, work outside the home is a financial necessity for growing numbers of women in both single-parent and two-parent households.

The benefits of work are many, but certain occupations co-exist with serious hazards, stemming from our shameful history of considering the worker as a "thing"—literally true during the age of slavery and virtually true during the Industrial Revolution. Industrial accidents and epidemics of lead poisoning and silicosis scarred the first part of this century; pockets of similar troubles exist to this day. Women

died horrific deaths as garment workers in the
Triangle Shirtwaist fire of 1911, in which 140 New
York City sweatshop workers were killed in the space
of a few minutes. Eighty years later, 25 poultry
processors were killed in the Imperial Foods fire in
Hamlet, North Carolina. Both tragedies involved
poor, mostly female workers; blocked safety exits;
and in the former, abysmal or no regulations, and, in
the latter, disregard for regulations. Both were entire-
ly preventable. Women in "pink collar" activities
experience hazards from neglect and abuse, while
those entering traditionally male fields have faced
hostility and inflexible workplace designs.

Occupational hazards are, by definition, the
result of human activity. The creative solutions to
overcoming them will also be the result of careful,
energetic human activity. What, then, are the health
and safety hazards women face as workers, and what
are the social, economic, and biological issues contributing to these problems? What health and safety
resources are available, and what resources need to
be developed?

WORKPLACE HAZARDS

Workplace problems are not exclusively gender identified; similarly, solutions will benefit both sexes.
Smaller-size safety equipment designed for women
will benefit smaller men; on-site day-care facilities
will benefit fathers as well as mothers. Nevertheless,

there are areas that disproportionately affect women and problems that are recognized only when women enter the labor force in substantial numbers. The three major issues are those based on size and shape differences, those concerning reproduction and pregnancy (some of which fall into the "size and shape" category), and those stemming from social factors. Women encounter these problems whether they work in traditional women's jobs or in jobs previously reserved for men.

The general differences in physical design and strength between men and women are the easiest to address. Traditionally, activities requiring occasional bursts of extreme physical strength have been separated from those requiring repetition or dexterity (hunting versus gathering, if you will). If you walk through an average manufacturing plant, you'll probably see areas of assembling or packaging where women are using small amounts of force with great frequency. Nearby there may be several men lifting boxes, hauling equipment, or resting during the slack time between the need for less frequent but more force-requiring activity. Needless to say, the chances are good that the men are paid nearly twice what the women are paid.

What about the old argument that each gender is doing what suits it best? The average man does have greater lifting capacity than the average woman, but there is considerable overlap across the male and female population. Furthermore, since lower back injuries are directly proportional to the lifting requirements of the job—and since they represent the single greatest work-related injury expense—better engi-

neering to minimize these requirements makes obvious sense. When the need for sporadic strength is less
predictable (during fire fighting or policework, for
example), then specific strength requirements must
be defined and applied equally to women and men.
The Americans with Disabilities Act of 1992 strictly
limits the use of physical requirements in job place-
ment. The requirements must legitimately reflect the
needs of the job, and there has to be no reasonable
way to alleviate the job's strength requirements.

The reverse argument, that women were some-
how better suited for repetitive handwork, has result-
ed in a massive wave of upper-extremity repetitive
strain injury, including carpal tunnel syndrome (pain
or numbness from pressure on the nerve passing
through the wrist) and a variety of types of tendonitis
(inflammation of the tissue that connects muscle to
bone). This type of injury now threatens to exceed
back injury as the most expensive work-related
injury, because it is no longer confined to factories
but is seen among clerical workers who spend entire
workdays glued to their computer keyboards. The
abuse of physical capabilities is unacceptable for
either men or women and cannot substitute for proper work process design.

What design changes are needed? Machine controls; operating heights; reach distances; and safety
equipment such as masks, goggles, and gloves must
be made to accommodate the range of body types in
the population. Women who work in traditionally
male industries often have to deal with ill-fitting gear
that may actually increase rather than decrease hazards. Women who work in traditionally female fields,

on the other hand, are assumed to have no safety problems and thus are generally ignored. This is foolish, since ergonomics (including the science of adapting the workplace to the worker) has shown us how to increase not only safety but also efficiency. As in any engineering field, new designs for the workplace require careful planning, and there must be prototype trials to ensure that the designs are safe and effective. What's more, subsequent monitoring under actual use is required to make sure the designs remain helpful. American industry's failure to attend to safe equipment design affects the entire work force, but its impact is greatest on women. (See Fig. 4.1).

There are other differences between men and women that are assumed to affect where women work and at what. Women have a different body composition, with a higher proportion of fat to muscle, and hips and elbows that are angled slightly differently from men's. Women also have a keener sense of smell. Some studies have shown slight gender-based differences in heat tolerance and stamina as well as in absorption, metabolism, and storage of some chemicals. None of these differences is absolute, and men and women outside the "average" range will overlap.

Furthermore, by law in this country each worker is entitled to a safe and healthful workplace. There are mandated margins of safety for exposures to chemical, biological, and physical hazards, and trivial differences between men and women should not matter. In areas in which such differences might be important, such as space exploration, women would be favored more often as not.

Nowhere are the problems of workplace safety and health more emotionally charged than when childbearing is discussed. Historically, the social and public health and reform movements that ended child labor and other abuses saw women also as victims. Hence, women were covered under protective

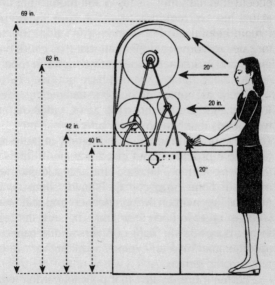

Figure 4.1.   A Well-Designed Work Station
Research in the field of ergonomics—the science of adapting the workplace environment to the physical attributes of the worker—has focused increasing attention on the safety and comfort of work stations. Critical angles and heights are taken into account in relation to the worker in the design of an ergonomic work station.

legislation. It was only after pressure from the women's movement, in fact, that some states removed restrictions on night work or double shifts for women.

Today, there is an increasing concern for the health of developing fetuses. Curiously, this concern is exhibited only when women attempt to enter traditionally male work areas and never seems to take into account the economic needs of the mother or child. No one has ever seriously argued that we bar women of reproductive age from working in child-care settings, where the risk of infections that may cause birth defects and miscarriage (such as measles and rubella) is quite real. Similarly, women have not been barred from work as nurses or hospital technicians, even though they may be exposed to gases, radiation, and medications that can adversely affect pregnancy.

The issues of pregnancy and fertility in the workplace have brought about court actions. In the late 1970s, the Oil, Chemical, and Atomic Workers Union sued the American Cyanamid Company on behalf of five women who underwent surgical sterilization in order to keep their jobs. They lost the case; the courts upheld the right of American Cyanamid to require women in lead-exposed work areas to document surgical sterility. And it wasn't until 1991 that the U.S. Supreme Court ruled that policies barring fertile women from a work area are discriminatory.

What are the issues here? Certainly no one wants knowingly to expose her child to poisons. But such poisons can affect men as well and have been shown to cause infertility and cancer in men and fetal deformity and cancer in their offspring. Policies that focus exclusively on women fail to protect children fully because they ignore critical paternal factors. Furthermore, these policies deny a woman control over her own reproduction and prevent her from making choices in her own or her family's best interests. The demise of women-focused policies will allow standards that minimize toxic exposures to everyone.

Of course, there are legitimate circumstances in which both women and men considering having a child may want to take greater precautions at work. For example, no one should have to tolerate the lead levels currently permitted in factories and construction by the Occupational Safety and Health Administration's (OSHA's) standards. But the risks to adults are considerably less than to children born of those adults, since exposure affects sperm, crosses the placenta, is excreted in breast milk, and targets the fetus's developing nervous tissue. The answer, however, is not to sterilize all workers in these industries but rather to encourage flexibility, such as allowing lateral transfers to nonexposed areas for workers starting a family. Many hospitals allow nurses and pharmacists to avoid mixing chemicals when pregnancy is planned, for example. It would be better to use special equipment to minimize everyone's exposure, because many chemicals that damage the developing fetus may also cause cancer in adults.

There are pregnancy workplace issues as well. At one time, women who worked outside the home were expected to resign when pregnant for social and cultural reasons. We know now that pregnant women can safely engage in moderate activity up to the time of delivery. On the other hand, some pregnant women entering the skilled trades have been subjected to an all-or-nothing approach to their work performance. Reasonable modifications can be made to accommodate the physical demands of pregnancy. As the center of gravity and balance changes later in pregnancy, climbing and lifting requirements need to be altered. Metabolic demands may require activity modification and may limit the use of respirators and other protective gear.

These accommodations are reasonable, yet they—and adequate maternity leave—are contested by some employers and co-workers, especially in the traditionally male professions and the blue-collar trades. We should see our children as a societal resource and responsibility. When the child arrives, parents have new concerns. Adequate leave for mother and/or father; good, safe, reliable child care; and ease and acceptability of breast-feeding are important issues for parents. To work full-time and to breast-feed with no supplemental formula feedings require enormous effort; a woman needs both privacy and time during the workday to express milk. This can be nearly impossible in many job settings, particularly industrial ones.

Another breast-feeding concern is toxic substances in the milk. A number of known hazards, such as lead and PCBs (a chemical now banned but once used in paints, in adhesives, as a machinery lubricant, and as an insulator), may enter the milk from storage sites in bone and fat or from ongoing exposure. If there are serious concerns, breast milk can be analyzed for toxic substances. The benefits of breast-feeding are overwhelmingly clear, and women should discontinue breast-feeding only when toxic contaminants are confirmed.

Economics may be another issue. Because some employers have been inflexible concerning the need for maternity leave, child care, flexible shifts, and so on, women have been forced to drop in and out of the work force in response to the needs of their families. Some "women's work" is thus characterized by low pay and few or no chances for promotion. When women leave and reenter the work force, they lose seniority and benefits. In the past, it was expected that men's work would be subsidized by women willing to assume all household duties.

As women enter the work force, the stress of home management and conducting family affairs often escalates. The need to perform as parent, tutor, laundress, chauffeur, cook, and housekeeper as well as breadwinner may be the result of single parenthood, a negotiated distribution of responsibilities, or a simple need to keep the peace. Women may be unable to negotiate equitable sharing of family responsibilities or to identify and enlist sources of help and support, and so they end up tired and resentful.

The options available for each one of us to cope with balancing home and work may differ markedly, but options do exist. Children can perform meaningful chores if rewarded by an appreciative parent (who is not inclined to step in to do the task herself). Simple meals and housekeeping just sufficient enough to prevent the spread of disease may in fact be the price of sanity. The point is, each woman must decide where her priorities lie and which battles are worth fighting. If dirty windows depress you, you may get more benefit from paid housekeeping help than from a family vacation.

Men have been excluded from this discussion, not because they're exempt from these responsibilities but because it is a matter of individual choice how much any woman wishes to negotiate with her mate. We must learn to respect each other's decisions.

Physical violence most often occurs in the home and must not be tolerated under any circumstances. However, it can also be an occupational hazard and is the leading cause of on-the-job death for women. Women in traditional jobs, such as working in a store, and in less traditional ones, such as driving a bus, have been killed and injured in the line of work. For most of these crimes, the gender of the victim is immaterial, although some may involve sexual harassment or rape. The threat of violence disproportionately affects women. We need to respond to it with specific preventive measures. Safety issues, which affect men and women alike, include adequate lighting, security personnel, acrylic partitions, emergency call buttons, and training in self-defense.

Much more specific to women is the issue of sexual harassment, a form of physical and psychological violence. It is encountered in female and male settings. Occasional cases of vicious, concerted, criminal activity have been reported. It requires courage and self-confidence to report and stop sexual harassment, and the good news is that courageous, self-confident women are reshaping the face of American institutions from the military to industry to academia.

Women in the workplace can face an array of obstacles to safety, serenity, and success. While emotional and psychological obstacles to an ideal workplace may not seem quite as great a challenge as exposure to toxic chemicals or dangerous equipment, the danger is still real. Archaic values and institutions as well as emotional and psychological assaults not only can create an environment that overlooks or even fosters danger but can also create terrible stress, a threat to health and well-being that must be considered.

ON-THE-JOB RISKS

Men and women, for the most part, face the same hazards in the workplace. On-the-job risks can be categorized as safety hazards (those that cause injury) or health hazards (those that cause disease). This distinction isn't absolute, and some conditions, such as lower back pain, might be considered either an injury or a disease. (These categories were initially set up to address industrial accidents but now include other problems.)

Safety Hazards

Safety hazards cause injury and death in obvious, often dramatic ways. Less obvious is the fact that good safety engineering and careful administration and inspection can prevent most of these tragedies. The term *accident* implies that an occurrence is unforeseen. Actually, careful evaluation of the work-site not only can foresee such problems but can often eliminate them.

Accurate statistics of deaths due to trauma in the workplace are difficult to ascertain, because different sources of information give different results. But approximately 10,000 workers die on the job each year, while another 22 million lose work because of a work-related injury (ranging in severity from mild sprains to permanent total impairment). Men greatly outnumber women in occupational mortality statistics, since they predominate in the more dangerous industries of mining, construction, and heavy-equipment operation. However, women who have entered these fields over the last 20 years have died these same preventable deaths. Because young workers are injured and killed disproportionately, the impact of this loss is far greater than the numbers themselves indicate. If we consider years of life lost (using the standard life expectancy for those killed), trauma, including motor vehicle, falls, and workplace injuries, causes greater losses than either heart disease or cancer.

The leading cause of death on the job is motor vehicle accidents, involving workers who drive as a part of their job. A review of motor vehicle safety gives us an opportunity to look at the *hierarchy of controls* that safety experts bring into play whenever safety issues are addressed. The first, best-level of response to a known hazard is to eliminate it. With auto safety, this would mean finding another work process—for example, communicating by fax or tele-conference instead of traveling. The second level in the hierarchy is to substitute specific material or equipment, such as using the train instead of the automobile.

Since these solutions are often not feasible, the third choice for prevention—engineering control—becomes a very important one. This includes environmental engineering, such as safe roads with adequate lighting, entry ramps, and dividers, as well as safety engineering for the vehicles. Vehicle safety starts with design and materials and concludes with specific parts such as dashboards, steering columns, and airbags. The engineered parts must be tested for safety and efficacy; what's more, it's critical that there be follow-up evaluation under actual road conditions.

The last level of the hierarchy of controls involves protective devices that rely on individual cooperation and participation, such as wearing a seatbelt.

All occupational safety can be considered under this hierarchy of controls. Overall issues need to be considered first, such as whether a particular plant is safe enough to build (e.g., a nuclear power plant), and how far from housing or schools certain facilities need to be. Next, safety must be built into the design and materials of a plant as well as into each item of equipment. Each procedure that needs to be performed should also be examined in terms of safety. Scrupulous attention to detail, including railings, machine guards, lock-out procedures, routine inspection and maintenance, safety and fire drills, and housekeeping is part of a safe working environment.

As the old poster said, "Safety is no accident!" To ensure that a high safety standard is maintained, facilities need a joint labor-management committee to evaluate the working environment and to solve safety problems.

Mining, construction, and agriculture, for which environmental engineering is difficult, have extremely high death and disability rates. Yet, even in these industries, careful consideration of equipment design, administrative practices, job training, safe work practices, and appropriate personal protective equipment can improve work site safety. Personal equipment (safety shoes, goggles, etc.) must fit properly, should not interfere with the worker's ability to function and communicate, and should be comfortable. Anyone who has ever been required to wear such equipment can testify that there is enormous room for improvement.

Health Hazards

Health hazards are often less obvious than safety hazards; the diseases they cause may take years to develop and often resemble diseases of nonoccupational origin. Occupational exposures may cause disease, join with other factors in developing disease, or may simply exacerbate a preexisting disease. All of this makes it difficult to measure the exact number of deaths and disabling conditions brought about by health hazards in the workplace. Conservative estimates attribute approximately 5 percent of cancer deaths to workplace carcinogen exposure. Job-related deaths from respiratory failure, poisoning, and renal and liver failure bring the estimated annual death toll to around 200,000. The toll of nonfatal disease is much higher. Common complaints include repetitive musculoskeletal injury (carpal tunnel syndrome, tendonitis, and the like), noise-induced hearing loss, dermatitis (skin inflammations), asthma, headaches, and stress-related symptoms. These problems impede functioning at work and at home. They often require medical care and interfere with the joy of living.

Health hazards are organized into four broad categories: biologic, mechanical, physical, and chemical. Biologic hazards include workplace-acquired infections such as hepatitis B and allergies to materials found at the job site. Mechanical hazards include repetitive lifting, pushing, pulling, and carrying as well as movements that require the individual to use awkward postures with varying degrees of force and repetition. Physical hazards consist of heat, cold, noise, vibration, light, high and low ambient air pressures, and various forms of radiation. Chemical hazards are ubiquitous in our workplaces and include both natural and synthetic substances such as solvents, metals, caustics, pesticides, catalysts, and acids.

In general, we need to consider whether a worker is actually being exposed to harmful substances and if it is possible to isolate the worker from such substances. Biologic and chemical hazards usually enter the body through breathing, swallowing, and/or skin absorption. Clouds of fine particles from grinding and heating (as when welding or burning) are inhaled. Workers who have inadequate hand-washing facilities or who eat or smoke at their work stations may ingest toxic material. Some substances are absorbed readily through the skin. For all categories of hazards we speak of a *dose-response* relationship. Within a normal range of variation and depending on the substance, there seems to be a connection between the amount of a substance a worker is exposed to and the severity of the symptoms or disease that results.

Disease can be prevented in much the same way accidents can. Safer procedures and substances can be substituted, as in agricultural practices that eliminate the need for pesticides and the use of fiberglass or rock wool insulation instead of asbestos. It is important to determine that the new substance doesn't have problems of its own, as has been the worry with fiberglass.

Engineering controls are also extremely important for disease prevention. Industrial hygienists—the engineers who usually address health hazards in the workplace—measure noise, chemicals, and other potential problems and design and implement machine modifications to protect the worker. Examples include soundproofing the booth a machine operator works in and installing exhaust ventilation close to a welding or grinding operation. Similarly, ergonomists evaluate mechanical hazards and develop and monitor means for preventing diseases such hazards can cause. The sources of safety problems that affect both men and women aren't limited to the factory floor.

No discussion of workplace hazards would be complete without mentioning child labor—still a fact of life throughout the world. In the United States child labor problems are evident in apparently innocuous jobs such as working in a fast-food restaurant. In many of these facilities, improper safety standards expose our teenage children to burns and worse. Children are killed working on farms, where machinery can be frighteningly complex and is underregulated. Certain marginal industries, particularly ones that rely heavily on illegal aliens, also hire children.

YOUR LEGAL RIGHTS AND RESOURCES

You have a legal right to work in a place and in a manner that is safe and healthy. Some threats to this, such as blocked exits, may be obvious, will affect everyone who works with you, and are regulated. Other problems, such as allergies to office indoor air pollution that is worse than established standards, may appear to be unique to you. You will have to rely on your own instincts and observations about what you can change yourself (making sure to choose the safest possible car if you're in sales, for example) and what will require outside intervention.

Depending on your circumstances, there are many avenues to pursue in search of relief of workplace dangers or of health problems you suspect are work-related (see "Where to Go for Help"). You can turn to both government and private agencies for help in correcting and preventing occupational hazards.

Government programs for occupational safety and health include federal, state, and local governments, with most of the resources being federal. OSHA was created by the Occupational Safety and Health Act of 1970. It is part of the Department of Labor and is charged with developing and enforcing regulations to ensure that every U.S. employee works in a safe and healthy environment.

Although the law says that the right to a safe and healthful workplace is absolute, in practice this right is often compromised. Employers balance workers' rights against financial considerations. Supreme Court rulings have instructed OSHA to demonstrate the cost/benefit ratio of new regulations; improvements in work environments are usually restricted to what is feasible and what will not cause industry undue hardship.

Complicating things still further, the process of setting standards is slow. Public hearings on proposed regulations are held, and some of the presented ideas are then incorporated into the final standard. And once regulations are established, they are frequently challenged in court. Moreover, groups of workers, such as those employed by small businesses (less than 10 employees), domestic workers, agricultural workers, construction workers, and government employees, are exempt from part or all of OSHA protection. Some OSHA regional offices, however, implement the "general duty" clause when a more specific regulation is lacking. This clause requires that employers have a general duty to provide a safe and healthful workplace. A number of states have developed their own plans that may be substituted for OSHA's as long as basic federal requirements are met.

OSHA has recently begun to focus on hospital safety and health, which is important because of concern about bloodborne diseases and multiply resistant tuberculosis. Standards exist for bloodborne disease transmission and use of ethylene oxide and formaldehyde (disinfectants and preservatives).

Repetitive strain injury has also been targeted by OSHA. The musculoskeletal complaints associated with computers are more difficult to address. Some obvious adjustments in seating, posture, arm, and screen heights can be made. The federal government says that the number of people with these injuries may be as high as 282,000. In response, OSHA is initiating proceedings to create regulations requiring all employers, including those in office settings, to do more to prevent these repetitive strain disorders.

The worst office environment is likely to have fewer measurable toxic exposures than most industries, even during office renovation. However, because of the nature of office work, even these levels of exposure may produce symptoms. Paint thinner can cause headaches, and nose and throat irritation, for example. Cigarette smoke is another irritant often found in the office building.

Hazard Communication gives workers the right to know about any potentially hazardous materials in the workplace. The standard requires employers to arrange training and to keep copies of a *Material Safety Data Sheet* (MSDS) for each potentially hazardous material at the job site. MSDSs list the specific chemical names for materials and emergency and toxicity information. They are provided by the manufacturers and distributors and may be kept in the purchasing department or in the company's safety office. If you are concerned about an exposure at work or have an illness that may be work related, ask for an MSDS for each substance you work with. Your doctor or your union health and safety specialist can independently check on the health effects of the chemicals. The manufacturer's contact number is also provided on ths MSDS, along with a 24-hour hot line number to call in case of emergency spills. In case of a spill, the emergency response team or physician will be able to call the manufacturer directly and speak with a chemist or toxicologist so that proper medical attention can be provided.

IMPROVING THE WORKPLACE

Your workplace is a significant part of your life; what goes on there can affect your health in equal measure. Occupational health and safety is your right and the right of every working woman. Know your rights and resources, but be aware that those resources may be limited. The workplace is already better because of our input. We need to work both individually and together to make sure that improvements continue to be made.

WHERE TO GO FOR HELP

Association of Occupational and Environmental Clinics (AOEC). AOEC can refer you to the nearest clinic so that your work-related health problem can be attended to. It can be reached at 202-347-4976, Monday through Friday, 9:00 A.M. to 5:00 P.M., Eastern Time.

CHEMTREC. CHEMTREC operates a hotline (800-262-8200) to assist the general public with nonemergency health, safety, and environmental questions about chemical products. It also distributes *Material Safety Data Sheets,* which include information about particular chemicals that workers may be exposed to. The hotline is open Monday through Friday, 9:00 A.M. to 6:00 P.M., Eastern Time.

Equal Employment Opportunity Commission (EEOC). EEOC will discuss, or help you file a report on, workplace challenges to your health and well-being from any kind of discrimination, including sexual harassment. It can be reached 24 hours a day at 800-669-4000.

National Institute for Occupational Safety and Health (NIOSH). Part of the Center for Disease Control, NIOSH was set up to research occupational health and safety. If you have an unusual problem or one that OSHA cannot address call the institute at 800-356-4674. NIOSH can inspect a work site and make recommendations but has no enforcement powers. It can provide information on a variety of subjects and has a continuing education program.

Occupational Health and Safety Administration (OSHA). OSHA can inspect and enforce workplace safety regulations. It also offers free consultations to small businesses. Look in the government section of your telephone book under "Department of Labor" or "Labor Department."

Office of Occupational Medicine. The Office of Occupational Medicine is an OSHA consulting service for physicians who want more detailed information about an occupational illness or injury. You may want to mention this service to your doctor. It can be reached at 202-219-5003, Monday through Friday, 8:00 A.M. to 5:00 P.M., Eastern Time.

Union. Find out if your union has a health and safety officer. That person may know of other local, national, and international resources.

Workers Compensation. Workers compensation provides income support and medical expenses for workers disabled by work-related injury or illness. It may offer help if your problem is not yet regulated or you have problems that fall under official guidelines. Look in the government section of your telephone book under "Department of Labor" or "Labor Department."

EDITORS AND CONTRIBUTORS

MEDICAL CO-EDITORS

ROSELYN PAYNE EPPS, M.D., M.P.H., M.A., F.A.A.P., is an expert at the National Institutes of Health, Bethesda, Maryland, and a Professor at Howard University College of Medicine, Washington, D.C. She is recognized nationally and internationally in areas of health policy and research, health promotion and disease prevention, and medical education and health service delivery. As a pioneer and leader in numerous professional and community organizations, she served, in 1991, as the first African-American president of AMWA and the founding president of the AMWA foundation.

SUSAN COBB STEWART, M.D., F.A.C.P., is an internist and gastroenterologist, and is presently Associate Medical Director at J. P. Morgan in New York, where she delivers general medical care, specialty consultations, and preventive services. She is Clinical Assistant Professor of Medicine at SUNY, Brooklyn. Since serving as President of AMWA in 1990, Dr. Stewart has continued to help AMWA shape and focus its mission in the area of women's health.

CONTRIBUTORS

Diane L. Adams, M.D., M.P.H., is the medical officer in the Office of Science and Data Technology, U.S. Agency for Health Care Policy and Research. She is also an Associate Professor at the University of Maryland, Eastern Shore. Her research activities have focused on occupational and environmental health, rural health, and minority and women's health.

Elaine Bossak Feldman, M.D., F.A.C.P., is Professor Emerita of Medicine and Physiology and Endocrinology and Chief Emerita of the Section of Nutrition at the

Medical College of Georgia in Augusta. In addition, she is Director Emerita at the Georgia Institute of Human Nutrition and a former member of the Bureau of Scientific Counselors of the National Cancer Institute.

Janet Emily Freedman, M.D., is the Acting Medical Director of Rehabilitation Medicine at Bellevue Hospital in New York. She is Assistant Professor of Rehabilitation Medicine at New York University Medical Center.

Rosemary K. Sokas, M.D., M.O.H., F.A.C.P., is an Associate Professor of Medicine and of Health Care Sciences at George Washington University in Washington, D.C., where she directs the Environmental/Occupational Health Program and the Occupational Medicine Residency Program.